ILLICIT DRUG USE:
Acute and chronic pharmacological intervention

This document was compiled on behalf of and in conjunction with the North West Anglia Healthcare Trust, Community Drugs Team, by Jonathan C Beard, BPharm, MSc, Dip (Clin.Pharm) MRPharmS. Mr Beard is a Senior Pharmacist employed by the Peterborough Hospitals NHS Trust.

ILLICIT DRUG USE:
Acute and chronic pharmacological intervention

by
Jonathan C Beard

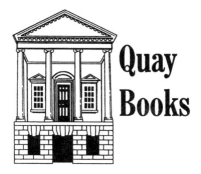

Quay Books

Quay Books Division of Mark Allen Publishing Limited
Jesses Farm, Snow Hill, Dinton
Salisbury, Wiltshire, SP3 5HN

British Library Cataloguing-in-Publication Data
A catalogue record is available for this book

© Mark Allen Publishing Limited, 1995
ISBN 1 85642 136 8

Printed and bound in Great Britain by
Biddles Limited, Guildford and King's Lynn

CONTENTS

Contents

ACKNOWLEDGEMENTS

I would like to thank the following people for their support, guidance and constructive criticism during the compilation of this document:

Mrs Meg Nicol RMN, Community Psychiatric Nurse
Mr Martin Alster RMN, Community Psychiatric Nurse
Dr Hugh Kilgour, Consultant Psychiatrist
Dr Dai Rowlands, Consultant Physician
Dr Robin Glover, Consultant in Accident and Emergency Medicine
Dr Simon Tuck, Consultant Paediatrician

I would also like to thank Miss Cheryl Coulson, Clerical Officer, for her extreme patience and secretarial assistance in compiling this document.

J C Beard

INTRODUCTION

This booklet evolved over a period of two years from a series of drug information queries posed by the North West Anglia Health Care Trust Community Drugs Team (CDT). Initially such queries involved a review of treatment strategies for opioid-dependent individuals and withdrawal syndrome management. However, a request to 'anglicise' a series of American protocols for treatment of acute illicit drug intoxication was the major determinant for the production of this booklet.

The compendium is unashamedly substance-orientated and aims to provide a detailed guide to the specific challenges resulting from drug use. The format is one of introduction followed by a description of both acute and chronic intoxication accompanied by various management options. Tolerance, dependence potential and relevant withdrawal syndromes are dealt with last and medical complications associated with any stage of illicit drug use are addressed in the appropriate section.

Each section concerned with the treatment of acute intoxication is prefaced with the warning that the information is for reference only and that all cases of acute substance intoxication should by referred to a National Poisons Information Centre for current management advice. This is to ensure that clients are not put at risk by the use of outdated information.

Numerous lists of signs/symptoms associated with intoxication and withdrawal are included. They are not arranged in any particular order unless otherwise stated but serve to show what might be encountered.

It is the CDT's hope that the information contained in this booklet will be of use to other health care professionals working in this area. Comments and ideas for change or updating will be gratefully received and should be directed to J C Beard, at the following address:

> Pharmacy Department
> Edith Cavell Hospital
> Bretton Gate
> PETERBOROUGH
> PE3 9GZ

Chapter 1
OPIOIDS

The term opioid has been used to describe a number of chemically distinct synthetic compounds with morphine-like pharmacology.

Morphine itself is derived from the plant species Papaver Somniferum (sleep bringer), or opium poppy and strictly speaking is an opiate. It is a secondary plant metabolite or alkaloid contained with others in the exudate from the scored, unripened poppy capsule; hence the word 'opium' which is derived from the latin 'opion' meaning 'juice'. Morphine was first chemically isolated in the early seventeenth century, its name being derived from that of Morpheus, the Greco-Roman deity of dreams. Currently the term opioid is taken to include morphine and its derivatives (the opiates).

Medicinally, opioids are used mainly for their analgesic properties. However, their pharmacology is complex and several endogenous opioid peptides have been identified including enkephalins and dynorphins. They are believed to be in some way involved in behaviour and mood regulation. Their effects are mediated through interactions with specific endogenous opioid receptors located in various parts of the body, including areas of the brain, such as the thalamus, hypothalamus, midbrain, striatum, spinal cord and limbic system. These opioid receptors have been subdivided into mu, kappa, delta, sigma and epsilon types.

Exogenous opioids have varying affinities for these receptors and exert their effect through them[1].

Desired effects of opioids

Correct medicinal uses of opioids are not associated with significant incidence of drug dependence and are unlikely to lead to illicit drug use. However, when potent opioids such as morphine or heroin (diamorphine) are intravenously injected or inhaled, the user will experience a powerful euphoria. This is followed by a warm feeling due to peripheral vasodilation and the user may report feelings of relaxation and contentedness.

Larger doses result in varying degrees of sedation. It is these perceptually pleasant effects that lead to illicit opioid consumption.

Unfortunately, chronic illicit opioid use leads to tolerance to the drug's effects and also physical and psychological dependence. Under such circumstances abrupt drug discontinuation will result in a characteristic withdrawal syndrome which may be severe. Continued drug use allows the user to avoid this withdrawal syndrome.

Substances that act at opioid receptors:

Agonists	Partial agonists	Antagonists
Alfentanil	Buprenorphine	Diprenorphine
Codeine	Butorphanol	Levallorphan
Dextromoramide	Meptazinol	Nalmefene
Dextropropoxyphene	Nalbuphine	Nalorphine
Diamorphine	Pentazocine	Naloxone
Dihydrocodeine		Naltrexone
Dipipanone		
Fentanyl		
Levomethadyl		
Methadone		
Morphine		
Pethidine		

Generally, opioid agonists and partial agonists produce dependence. However the opioid receptor antagonists nalorphine and levallorphan have also rarely been reported to do so [2]

Acute opioid intoxication

Opioid intoxication results in central nervous system depression ranging from stupor to coma. It may result from deliberate or accidental administration and affects both new and seasoned users.

Characteristics of acute intoxication

Common signs of intoxication are as follows:	
Respiratory depression progressing to cyanosis	Hypotension
Nausea and vomiting	Bradycardia
Cold clammy skin and hypothermia	Skeletal muscle flaccidity
Progression to unconsciousness and coma	'Pin point pupils' (miosis)

Rapid intravenous administration of large doses of opioids may produce the following effects:	
Apnoea	Circulatory collapse
Cardiac arrest	Respiratory arrest

Other rarer medical complications of intoxication include pneumonia, shock and pulmonary oedema. Miosis may be present but mydriasis (dilated pupils) may occur with severe hypoxia. Mydriasis is also a feature of Diconal intoxication. Since Diconal contains the antihistamine cyclizine which has antimuscarinic properties, acute intoxication with this preparation results in a mixture of antihistaminic, opioid and antimuscarinic effects. Cyclizine has recognised misuse potential being associated with euphoria and hallucinations when intravenously injected.

Pethidine has a degree of intrinsic antimuscarinic activity and so has certain peculiar acute intoxicant characteristics.

Signs and symptoms of acute intoxication with antimuscarinic preparations include the following:	
Mydriasis	Excitation
Dry mouth and mucous membranes	Increased muscular activity, tremor, twitching
Tachycardia	Delirium with disorientation
Hallucinations	Tonic-clonic seizures

Treatment of acute intoxication

The following information on acute opioid intoxication is for reference only. All cases of acute substance intoxication require referral to a National Poisons Information Centre for current management advice.

General management

- Contact a Poisons Centre for current advice
- Hospitalisation is necessary
- The patient should be kept conscious/aroused
- Changing the patient's position frequently is advisable
- Ensure the patient's airways are clear
- Respiration can be stimulated by a mixture of O_2 and 5% CO_2

Specific treatment

The signs and symptoms of opioid overdose may be reversed by administration of an opioid antagonist. However general interventions should not be neglected before antagonist therapy can be administered. Naloxone is the drug of choice and may be used as follows:

- Naloxone is administered at a dose of 0.4mg to 2mg intravenously which may be repeated at 2 to 3 minute intervals to a dose of 10mg if respiratory function does not improve. Subcutaneous or intramuscular routes should only be used when the intravenous route is unavailable (as in chronic intravenous drug users). Naloxone may be administered by continous intravenous infusion (2mg/500ml 0.9% sodium chloride) at a rate determined by response[3].

The infusion rate may be determined by noting the hourly naloxone requirements over the first three to four hours of therapy. It may then be adjusted to deliver that hourly rate[4]. It is important not to discharge overdose patients within 24 hours of treatment as the duration of action of naloxone is shorter than that of most opioids.

In some cases it may be necessary to use up to 20mg naloxone especially in cases of intoxication with codeine, dextropropoxyphene and fentanyl derivatives[4].

It is not necessary or desirable to precipitate opioid withdrawal syndrome in dependent individuals as the symptoms are more severe than when produced by abstinence alone. Aggression and excitation have been reported in such cases and patients may be very difficult to handle. The end point of therapy should be stabilisation of the patient's vital signs, by careful incremental naloxone administration.

Seizures may be associated with hypoxia secondary to respiratory depression and have also been reported with Diconal, dextropropoxyphene and pethidine intoxication.

Diconal (dipipanone and cyclizine) and pethidine are associated with antimuscarinic effects. Seizures may be managed by intravenous or rectal diazepam.

In the UK, dextropropoxyphene is formulated with paracetamol (co-proxamol) and it is important to treat both opioid and paracetamol poisoning in cases of co-proxamol overdose.

Opioid dependence

The illicit use of opioids leads to tolerance and dependence. However acute overdose is still a possibility. Tolerance to all of an opioid's effects is not always the case and pethidine users often exhibit its antimuscarinic effects. Chronic opioid use may result in certain behavioural and physical characteristics.

Characteristics of dependence

Behavioural:	
• Euphoria	• Drowsiness
• Nodding (known as gouching)	• Loss of appetite
• Loss of sexual drive	• Altered personality/activities
• Inattentiveness	

Physical:	
• Miosis (less with seasoned users, diconal and 'pethidine-like' opioids)	• Itching nose/skin
• Needle tracks on the body (extremities, groin, abdomen)	• Nausea and vomiting (less with seasoned users)
• Bradycardia (less with diconal and pethidine)	• Slowed respiration
• Constipation	

Diagnostic tests for dependence

The administration of an opioid antagonist in sufficient dose or abrupt opioid discontinuation in a dependent individual will precipitate a withdrawal syndrome. This can be extremely unpleasant and cannot be recommended as a diagnostic test.

However experimental use of two drops of 1mg/ml naloxone in 0.9% sodium chloride applied conjunctivally has been shown to demonstrate significant pupillary dilation in methadone maintained dependent individuals. Non-dependent subjects did not show the same response[5]. Whether this is a reliable test for opioid dependence remains to be seen. It was not reported as to whether the test worked in individuals who were using pethidine which has an intrinsic mydriatic effect.

Opioid withdrawal syndrome

Several weeks of continuous consumption of a potent opioid may be sufficient to cause physical dependence. However, this has been reported to be a minor problem when the opioid is used as an analgesic even at very large doses. Following abrupt discontinuation of opioids, the dependent individual will display a withdrawal syndrome. The onset, intensity and duration of the syndrome depends upon several factors including the opioid used, total daily dose, duration of use and personality of the user. Generally longer acting opioids produce milder but prolonged withdrawal effects whilst short acting agents produce more intense but shorter withdrawal effects.

Characteristics of opioid withdrawal syndrome

Opioid	Peak Withdrawal Symptoms (time after discontinuation)
Heroin (diamorphine)	36–48 hours
Morphine	36–72 hours
Pethidine	8–12 hours
Methadone	approx. 3–6 days

Signs and symptoms are as follows: [1,4 6,7,8]		
Running nose	Muscle twitch	Vomiting
Tremor	Kicking movements	Diarrhoea
Perspiration	Yawning	Lacrimation
Goose flesh	Sneezing	Mydriasis
Spasm	Spontaneous ejaculation	Anorexia
Increased body temperature		Nausea
Increased respiratory rate	Insomnia	Hot and cold flushes
Increased blood pressure	Muscle cramp	Restlessness
Increased heart rate	Muscular aching	
Raised urinary [17] ketosteroids		
Leukocystosis		
Craving		
Anxiety		

The combined effects of vomiting, diarrhoea, perspiration and anorexia can result in acute weight loss, dehydration, ketosis and acid-base and electrolyte imbalance. Cardiovascular collapse is a rare complication of peak severity withdrawal.

Drug treatments for opioid dependent individuals

Opioid-dependent individuals may seek help from health care workers either to obtain legal supplies of drugs or to stop opioid consumption altogether. Some health care workers view this scenario to be a forerunner to complete abstinence. However, this is not necessarily the case as the end point of therapy may be the avoidance of illegal opioids and the activities necessary to fund their acquisition. With this in mind, maintenance therapy may be required in some individuals for years, even life.

Discontinuation of opioids

The often extremely unpleasant withdrawal syndrome is one factor responsible for continued opioid use in the dependent individual. However the process of opioid withdrawal is reported to be easily achieved[9]. Equally, if not more important, is continued abstinence. This is reported to be very difficult for ex-dependants to maintain without effective social and psychological support from health care workers and others in the community[9,10].

Opioid discontinuation has been achieved by a number of methods. Simple abrupt discontinuation followed by withdrawal syndrome has been used but is usually not acceptable to the client. Gradual discontinuation is another approach, often first transferring to longer acting drugs such as methadone[10]. Gradually reducing the daily dose of methadone (a 'reducing script') attenuates the withdrawal syndrome making it more bearable.

Other methods of easing withdrawal discomfort involve the use of clonidine[11] or clonidine combined with naltrexone[8]. Indeed cocaine has been reported to reduce withdrawal syndrome severity but its use as a withdrawal adjunctive is probably not to be recommended.

Whichever withdrawal technique is used, flexibility is very important. Drop out rates from such programmes are high[9] and continued abstinence following successful withdrawal is often poor[12]. The dependency process is complex and ex-clients may require support and encouragement to avoid lapsing back into illicit use. One pharmacological approach is the use of the opioid antagonist, naltrexone[2,4], which may encourage abstinence.

Opioid dosage reduction ('the reducing script'): Dosage reduction regimens involve gradual decreases in a client's daily intake until opioid administration can be stopped. This 'weaning off' process reduces the intensity of the withdrawal syndrome to a more bearable level.

Any opioid may be used in dosage reduction regimens including morphine, heroin, buprenorphine and methadone. However, over the years methadone has gained prominence. It has the advantage of having a long duration of action, making it suitable for once daily administration[1]. It is also reported to block euphoriant effects of other opioids at high doses but this has been challenged[4].

When methadone is employed the first step in the process is to determine the clients daily opioid intake. An equivalent dose of methadone is then substituted for the illicit drug.

Methadone is equivalent to morphine on a mg per mg basis when administered acutely. However, chronic methadone administration leads to accumulation. As a guide, 1mg of methadone (administered chronically) is approximately equivalent to 2mg of diamorphine (pharmaceutical grade), 3–4mg of morphine, 20–25mg of pethidine, 0.04mg buprenorphine, 2–2.5mg of dipipanone, 10–12.5mg pentazocine and 15mg codeine. Clients' recall of their daily drug consumption may be faulted due to, among other things, the very variable purity of opioids obtained illicitly. Thus, one or two days may then be necessary to adjust this initial dose appropriately. McKinney*et al* reviewed three popular methadone dosage reduction regimens employed in various centres throughout the USA[4]. These are summarised as follows:

1. Once the equivalent methadone dose has been established the daily dose is reduced by 20 percent every day for ten days. Methadone is then discontinued.

2. Some practitioners do not advocate methadone doses in excess of 50mg daily. Methadone is introduced at a dose of 10mg four times daily and adjusted over two days. The adjusted dose is then reduced by 5mg daily until withdrawal is achieved.

   Clients requiring methadone doses less than 40mg have their dosage adjusted over two days. The methadone is then withdrawn in eight steps over eight days.

3. A five day withdrawal regimen is reported to have been developed and used by clients themselves. The initial daily methadone dose is 100mg regardless of the dependent individuals daily opioid intake. This dose is reduced by 50% as are subsequent doses until withdrawal is achieved ie.

100mg, 50mg, 25mg, 12.5mg, 6mg, stop.

These withdrawal regimens are fixed with little flexibility for dosage adjustment; the participating client is withdrawn from methadone over 5–12 days. Some practitioners involve a longer regimen taking three to four weeks or more to achieve detoxification[9].

With gradual methadone withdrawal regimens, clients experience withdrawal symptoms towards the end of the treatment regimen, and sometimes up to a month afterwards. Clients are usually relatively symptom free for the first few methadone decrements

Clonidine withdrawal therapy: The opioid withdrawal syndrome involves, in part, an increase in central nervous system activity particularly in an area called the *locus ceruleus*[11]. This increased CNS activity involves the neurotransmitter noradrenaline, explaining some of the 'stimulant' characteristics of the withdrawal syndrome, eg. increased blood pressure and heart rate, anxiety, restlessness and insomnia.

Clonidine is an alpha-2-adrenergic agonist which stimulates pre-synaptic (inhibitory) alpha-adrenergic receptors. This results in less noradrenaline release from the *locus ceruleus* and alleviation of some withdrawal symptoms.

Clonidine withdrawal therapy involves abrupt discontinuation of the client's opioids. The ensuing withdrawal syndrome is then attenuated by careful administration of clonidine

A suggested fourteen day clonidine withdrawal regimen is outlined below[11].

Day '1' represents the onset of the withdrawal syndrome. For short acting opioids Day 1 may be the day of abrupt discontinuation but a delay in withdrawal syndrome onset is expected with longer acting opioids.

Clonidine administration causes a mean blood-pressure drop of 10 to 15mm Hg. It has been suggested that clonidine should be withheld when systolic blood pressure falls below 85mm Hg. Monitoring a client's blood pressure regularly is therefore necessary.

Clonidine withdrawal regimen[11]

Day	Clonidine dose mcg/kg body weight	Administration times	
1	6	0800/2200	hours
2–10	7	0800/2200	hours
	3	1500	hours
11	3	0800	hours
	1	1500	hours
	4	2200	hours
12	2	0800/2200	hours
13	2	0800	hours
14	0	—	

This regimen has been used in the US and the UK but is only to be used as a guide. Clients may respond differently to a given clonidine dose requiring more or less to alleviate withdrawal effects and limit side-effects.

Clonidine side-effects include drowsiness, depression, fluid retention, headache, dizziness, constipation, hypotension, Raynaud's phenomenon and insomnia [13]. Insomnia has been successfully managed with long acting benzodiazepines such as flurazepam (which is NHS blacklisted) and nitrazepam. Its management should not be neglected as insomnia is a major reason for failing to complete such regimens. Hypotension can be easily managed by clonidine dose reduction whilst severe hypotension may require further specialist medical treatment. Abrupt discontinuation of clonidine has resulted in rebound hypertension. This can be successfully managed by reintroduction of clonidine followed by more gradual withdrawal but is unlikely to be a problem with a fourteen day regimen.

Muscle pain/discomfort associated with withdrawal may be managed using paracetamol or non-steroidal anti-inflammatory agents. Diazepam has also been used in this respect.

Psychotic reactions have been reported in patients using clonidine to withdraw from opioids[8,11]. Patients with previous mental illness may be predisposed to this.

When compared to methadone dosage reduction, results are similar but withdrawal distress is worst in the first few days of clonidine therapy rather than later as with methadone reduction. As clonidine therapy results in marked hypotension and insomnia this method of withdrawal is managed in hospital. Also, clonidine is not licensed for this indication.

Lofexidine withdrawal therapy: Lofexidine is a clonidine-analogue with reportedly less sedative and hypotensive potential than clonidine itself[14]. It is licensed for the relief of symptoms of patients undergoing opioid dextoxification. The initial dose is 0.2mg orally twice daily. This may be increased in increments of 0.2–0.4mg daily up to 2.4mg per day. The duration of therapy is recommended to be 7 to 10 days after abrupt opioid discontinuation[15]. Being less sedative and hypotensive than clonidine, it has been investigated for outpatient use as regular blood pressure monitoring is not crucial[14,16]. The cost of the therapy is very high in comparison to clonidine, but must be viewed in the context of intended outpatient therapy. Its lack of side-effects are preferred by clients and staff. Other withdrawal symptoms can be managed as outlined in the section on clonidine-naltrexone withdrawal therapy.

Clonidine-naltrexone withdrawal therapy: With this method of opioid discontinuation, the clonidine is used to attenuate the withdrawal syndrome whilst naltrexone is used to precipitate the syndrome more rapidly. Used alone in an opioid dependent individual naltrexone, (a long-acting opioid antagonist) would rapidly induce withdrawal. Such an antagonist induced withdrawal is very intense but of a shorter duration than of one produced by abstinence alone. Hence, clonidine and naltrexone are used to achieve opioid discontinuation in four to five days. The shorter regimen represents a very significant saving when compared to methadone reduction therapy assuming both are performed in the hospital setting. Charney *et al* reported successful withdrawal of 38 out of 40 methadone-dependent individuals using combined clonidine and naltrexone therapy.

Withdrawal was rapidly achieved in four to five days[8]. The clonidine-naltrexone regimen used is outlined below

Methadone day: This was the last day of normal methadone maintenance. No more methadone was administered unless intolerable withdrawal symptoms or hallucinations occurred (The methadone dose was about 40–50mg daily, sometimes higher).

Clonidine-naltrexone day 1: Clonidine was administered orally at a starting dose of 5mcg/kg at 9am. Two subsequent doses were given at 3pm and 9pm. The dose size was determined by withdrawal symptoms and clonidine side-effects.

Naltrexone was administered as follows:		
1 mg	orally	9 am
2 mg	orally	1 pm
3 mg	orally	5 pm
3 mg	orally	9 pm

Clonidine-naltrexone day 2: Clonidine was administered as on clonidine-naltrexone day 1

Naltrexone was administered as follows:	
5mg	9am
7mg	1pm
9mg	5pm
9mg	9pm

Clonidine-naltrexone day 3: Clonidine was administered three times daily as required.

Naltrexone was administered as follows:
10mg @ 9am, 1pm, 5pm
10–15mg @ 1pm

Clonidine-naltrexone day 4

> Clonidine was administered three times daily as required
>
> Naltrexone was administered as 50mg in the morning or as divided doses throughout the day

On the fifth day of the regimen the patients were discharged on sufficient naltrexone to block the effects of exogenous opioids. Clonidine was also dispensed to be used if necessary.

A second approach to rapid opioid withdrawal using clonidine and naltrexone was outlined by Haygarth[17], and has been used with success at High Royds Hospital, West Yorkshire. It is summarised as follows:

Day 1: Opioids were discontinued and the client given an oral trial dose of clonidine 0.1mg. BP measurements were taken 30 minutes, one and two hours after administration to assess clonidine's hypotensive potential.

A second oral clonidine dose was given provided hypotension was not marked and further doses were administered at four to six hourly intervals according to need and the following BP criteria:

BP (mm Hg)	Clonidine
>110/60	0.3 mg
110/60–100/60	0.2 mg
100/60–95/60	0.1 mg
Systolic < 95	0

Day 2: Clonidine was given orally as required according to the BP criteria. Other symptoms were controlled as follows:

- Hypersecretions and gastrointestinal hyperactivity — hyoscine butylbromide 20mg orally up to four times daily

- Anxiety — diazepam orally up to 80mg daily

- Diarrhoea — Lomotil (Co-phenotrope) orally up to

four times daily.

- Night sedation — Chloral hydrate 0.5–1g or nitrazepam 10mg orally at night

Day 3: Clonidine was given orally as required and symptoms treated as on day 2. The client was challenged with a 400mcg intramuscular naloxone injection. Clients with minimal withdrawal symptoms were given naltrexone 12.5mg orally.

Day 4: Clonidine was given as required and symptoms treated as on day 2. Clients were given a single 25mg naltrexone dose orally.

Day 5: Clonidine was given as required and symptoms treated as on Day 2. Clients were given a single oral 50mg naltrexone dose if symptoms allowed.

The regimen of clonidine 'as required', symptom control and naltrexone (50mg daily) were maintained until withdrawal symptoms subsided. Hospital discharge was considered on day[7].

Naltrexone and opioid abstinence

Naltrexone is a long-acting opioid antagonist and a 100mg oral dose can block the effects of exogenous opioids for up to 48 hours. Once a client has achieved abstinence naltrexone can be given to block the desired effects of opioids should they start to use them again. Initiation of the regimen involves an intravenous naloxone challenge, to ensure the client is indeed opioid abstinent before giving naltrexone. Assuming the naloxone test is uneventful, naltrexone therapy can be started at 25mg daily for a week followed by 50mg daily. A convenient regimen to achieve week long opioid antagonism is 100mg oral naltrexone on Mondays and Wednesdays and 150mg on Fridays. Clients should be warned not to attempt to overcome the 'block' with large opioid doses as potentially fatal intoxication may ensue.

Methadone maintenance therapy

Methadone is commonly used as a legal substitute for illicit opioids. This technique for treating clients has been criticised heavily in the past on both moral and technical grounds[12]. However it has recently regained favour.

The aim of maintenance therapy is to legally supply opioid dependent clients with sufficient opioids to suppress any desire to obtain illicit supplies. Methadone is used as it has a long duration of action and can be given orally daily. Such treatment is reported to have several advantages for clients, their associates and the community. These are as follows:

1. Reduced drug-related crime[18]

2. Reduced urge to obtain opioids so encouraging social and recreational rehabilitation[18]

3. Reduced chances of contracting HIV, Hepatitis B and C viruses via intravenous administration of illicit opioids using contaminated equipment

4. A reduced rate of progression to AIDS in already HIV seropositive opioid dependent individuals[19]

5. Improved social status. e.g. employment, improved relationships, improved child care and finances

6. Increased contact with community drug agencies and primary health care

7. Decreased overall mortality and morbidity.

Methadone is not popular with all recipients some of whom complain that it causes weight gain and bad teeth [20]. It is also reported to have an inferior euphoric affect and some clients prefer agents such as dihydrocodeine or codeine linctus.

There has also been interest in the use of buprenorphine as a 'maintenance opioid' [18] although it is also widely misused[21,22]. Methadone maintenance therapy may not be entirely free of significant risks. It has been suggested that methadone use in opioid dependent clients with chronic persistent hepatitis may lead to fatalities [23] and that lower initial doses should be used in such individuals.

Recent work suggests that about 80% of opioid dependants can be satisfactorily maintained on between 40 to 50mg of methadone daily [24]. Rarely, individuals may require more methadone and daily doses of 200mg are not unknown[10]. Generally doses should be no higher than those found to suppress symptoms in the client concerned.

Where part of the dependency is associated with the ritual of injecting, methadone has been administered intravenously using the contents of 35mg/3.5ml, 50mg/5ml, 10mg/ml or 50mg/ml methadone ampoules. These products are manufactured for intramuscular or subcutaneous administration and the contents are not isotonic with plasma. This has led to some clients experiencing a more rapid sclerosing of injected veins.

Clients should be warned that intravenous administration is not the intended route for such products.

Other opioids tried in maintenance therapy

Levomethadyl acetate: Levomethadyl acetate (LAAM) is a drug that is metabolised to long-acting opioid agonists in the body. It was developed in the 1940s as an analgesic but was found to be unsuitable because of its long onset of action. It was investigated in the 1970s and early 1980s as a potential maintenance opioid but did not become established for this purpose. However, resurgence of opioid maintenance therapy in the USA led to the FDA granting a licence for the use of LAAM as a maintenance opioid in 1993.

The potential advantages of LAAM are as follows:

1. On intravenous administration there is no opioid euphoria as the drug requires metabolism to become active. This markedly reduces its potential for illicit use

2. Its long duration of action allows for thrice weekly administration

3. On discontinuation, the associated withdrawal syndrome is milder than that associated with methadone.

Buprenorphine: The partial agonist buprenorphine has been investigated for its use in opioid dependency. Johnson *et al*[25,26] reported introducing buprenorphine to diamorphine dependent individuals at an initial dose of 2mg sublingually. This dose was doubled on two consecutive days to the final maintenance dose of 8mg sublingually. The opioid dependent individuals involved are reported to have received the buprenorphine very favourably.

Diamorphine: Diamorphine has been investigated as a maintenance opioid. Users are apparently unable to distinguish between it and methadone when it is administered orally.

In 1990, Marks and Palombella reported the use of diamorphine impregnated cigarettes (reefers) sometimes used in conjunction with oral stimulants[20]. This practice was said to produce the intense, immediate euphoria of intravenous opioid use without the concomitant risks of injections. The authors also stated that heroin reefers had less dependence potential than oral methadone thus facilitating easier discontinuation.

In 1994, the Royal Pharmaceutical Society issued an approved protocol for the preparation, storage, and recording of supply of diamorphine reefers from hospital and community pharmacies. The usual diamorphine content of each reefer is 60mg as the hydrochloride salt, but other drugs can also be incorporated into such reefer.

Chapter 2
CENTRAL NERVOUS SYSTEM STIMULANTS

As their name suggests, central nervous system stimulants excite the CNS. They do this by increasing the levels of excitatory neurotransmitters (eg. dopamine, noradrenaline, 5-hydroxytryptamine) in the neuronal synapses. This has the effect of augmenting normal neurotransmitter activity[27].

There are several naturally occuring potent CNS stimulants, the most well known being cocaine. The synthetic CNS stimulants are predominantly amphetamine analogues.

A list of common CNS stimulants is given below:

- Amphetamine/dexamphetamine (Dexedrine)

- Cocaine

- Dexfenfluramine (Adifax)

- Diethylpropion (Apisate, Tenuate Dospan)

- Fenfluramine (Ponderax)

- Mazindol (Teronac)

- Methylphenidate (Ritalin)

- Phentermine (Duromine/Lonamin)

CNS stimulants have few legitimate uses. They have been used as appetite suppressants and have been formally investigated for their potential to decrease fatigue and increase work output. Cocaine from the leaves of the coca plant, has been used by South American Indians for this purpose for centuries and was included in various tonic drinks in the past. Currently cocaine is used in the form of solution or paste as a local anaesthetic and vasoconstrictor in ENT surgery. It is also occasionally included as a constituent in 'The Bromptons Cocktail' although it is no longer recommended for this.

Methylphenidate has been used to treat hyperactive childen, and adults with attention deficit disorder have used illicit stimulants to ameliorate their symptoms reporting paradoxical calming effects.

CNS stimulants have the potential to produce feelings of wellbeing and alertness and, in certain circumstances, intense orgasmic euphoria.

The two main representatives of this group are cocaine and amphetamine both of which are widely used. They can cause habituation and dependence and in such circumstances abrupt discontinuation can result in a characteristic withdrawal syndrome.

Amphetamine and cocaine

Amphetamine is relatively easily and cheaply synthesised by individuals often with only a basic knowledge of chemistry. The final product may contain impurities with unpredictable effects. Their removal is more difficult than the initial synthesis and so is often not performed.

Amphetamine is usually ingested but can also be sniffed and injected. Reports of amphetamine-base smoking have also been documented in America[4]. The drug has a plasma half-life of between 6 and 24 hours being detectable in the blood for between 2 to 7 days after use. The desired euphoria lasts between 3 to 12 hours which is 4 to 8 times longer than that produced by cocaine.

Cocaine is extracted from the plant species Erythroxylum. It is available as the water soluble hydrochloride salt or as the free chemical base. The salt form is often adulterated with ephedrine (weak stimulant) and lignocaine (local anaesthetic). Cocaine base is more difficult to adulterate and is usually available in a high state of purity[4]. Cocaine hydrochloride is usually taken nasally (snorted) or administered intravenously, while cocaine base (also known as Crack, Freebase, Rock and Pasta) is vaporised by heating. The hot vapour is then inhaled or smoked. The speed at which the euphoriant effect takes place depends upon the administration route[27,28,29].

Route of Administration	Speed of Onset
Nasal	Up to 3 minutes
Intravenous	30–60 seconds
Inhalation (smoking)	5–10 seconds to 30 seconds

Cocaine has a plasma half-life of about 90 minutes with the euphoriant effect lasting for about 45 minutes, although this is less when smoked. Users demonstrate a rapidly developing tolerance to the effect even after the first dose. Repeated attempts to achieve the initial euphoria are unsuccessful and the dose administered has to be increased. This rapid tolerance is called tachyphylaxis (quick protection).

Patterns of CNS stimulant misuse

The following is applicable to both amphetamine and cocaine. The road to compulsive stimulant misuse is complex and only a small proportion of stimulant users progress to it. Figure 1 attempts to outline some common features.

Early stimulant use[27,28]

The new stimulant user usually starts with low doses. The result is that they experience increased alertness, wakefulness and a sense of wellbeing. Pleasurable experiences are reported to be magnified without distortion.

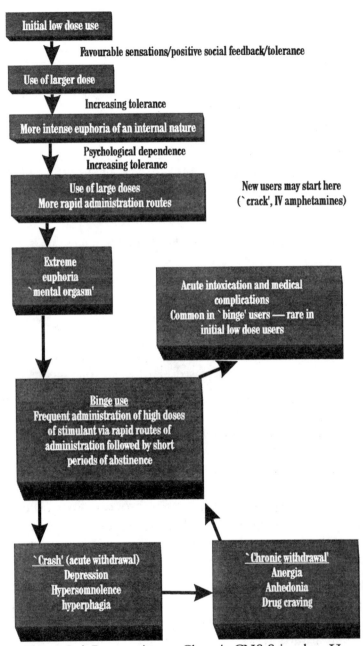

Figure 1 A Progression to Chronic CNS Stimulant Use

Characteristics of low dose CNS stimulant use in the new user[27,28]

- Undistorted magnification of pleasure
- Increased alertness
- Sensation of wellbeing
- Decreased anxiety
- Disinhibition
- Increased self-esteem, sociability and sexuality
- Decreased appetite
- Insomnia

Early low dose use results in favourable pharmacological effects and a positive social response. The user is thus encouraged to continue with this pleasurable and apparently harmless drug.

Transition to compulsive stimulant use[27,28,29]

Continued CNS stimulant use results in a very rapid development of tolerance (tachyphylaxis) to the effects of the drug. This tachyphylaxis causes the user to employ larger doses to achieve the desired effects. While experimenting with larger doses the user may experience a more intense drug-induced euphoria and begin to concentrate on this internal sensation while gradually withdrawing from stimulant use in the social setting.

The desire to repeatedly experience this internalised stimulant induced euphoria coupled with increasing tolerance and development of subsequent depression encourages continued use. Larger doses taken via rapid routes of administration (e.g. smoking cocaine, injecting amphetamines) results in euphoria so intense that it has been compared to an orgasm. Once experienced the CNS stimulant pattern of use is that of high doses, rapid administration routes and daily or 'binge' use.

CNS stimulant 'bingeing' [31]

'Binge' is a term used to describe a pattern of use involving frequent stimulant readministration over a relatively short time period.

The amphetamine 'binge' takes place over a period of days.

Chronic amphetamine users ('speed freaks') have been considered particularly unpredictable and dangerous, even by other illicit drug users[4]. This is a status currently held by Crack cocaine users. Cocaine bingeing involves readministration of the drug every 10 minutes or so up to 12 hours. Longer 'binges' have been reported.

Acute CNS stimulant intoxication

Acute intoxication with cocaine and amphetamine is indistinguishable, either to seasoned users, clinicians or laboratory animals. Acute intoxication is rare in low dose users but common with chronic high dose bingeing. In the uninitiated, small doses may cause severe intoxication and 10mg of amphetamine may be fatal to a child and 100mg to an adult. A 10mg dose of intravenous cocaine has proved fatal[30]. However chronic stimulant users may tolerate several grams of amphetamines or cocaine in a day as a result of progressive tachyphylaxis. Chronic stimulant use is also associated with certain medical complications

Characteristics of acute intoxication[27,28,29,31]

- Disinhibition
- Impaired judgement
- Grandiose ideas
- Impulsiveness
- Extreme wakefulness (hypervigilance)
- Markedly increased sexuality
- Feelings of superintelligence
- Rapid speech
- Compulsive repetitive actions (eg. picking at their skin)
- Aggression, restlessness, agitation
- Hallucinations recognised as being drug-induced
- Paranoid panic (fear of death)
- Paranoid psychosis with auditory hallucinations

- High dose induced spontaneous ejaculation
- Tremor/muscle contractions/exaggerated reflexes
- Tachycardia (rapid heart rate)
- Dry mouth/bad breath (chronic use)
- Hypertension (high blood pressure)
- Malnutrition (chronic use)
- Sweating
- Fever
- Dilated pupils
- Needle tracks (intravenous users)
- Palpitations
- Abnormal cardiac rhythms
- Abrupt involuntary movements and seizures
- Metabolic acidosis (cocaine)
- Low serum potassium levels
- Coma and circulatory collapse in fatal poisoning

Medical complications of high dose and chronic stimulant use

Medical complications of high dose and chronic stimulant use result mainly from vasoconstriction, cardiovascular stimulation and hypertension. Some problems are also associated with administration routes[4,27,29,31] and poor nutrition. Repeated daily injection of stimulants especially in a group setting, increases the risk of sharing injection equipment and transmission of blood born diseases e.g. Hepatitis, HIV.

Stimulants are sometimes used to enhance sexual pleasure ('speed sex') sometimes in a group setting and thus increases the risk of contracting or speading hepatitis, HIV and other sexually transmitted diseases.

Complications of snorting or smoking stimulants (cocaine)

- Nasal septum perforation
- CSF rhinorrhoea (cerebral spinal fluid leakage from the nose)
- Pulmonary oedema (fluid on the lungs)
- Pneumothorax (air accumulating in the pleural space)
- Pneumomediastinum (air accumulating in the tissue between the lungs)
- Chronic obstructive airways disease
- Headaches

Complications associated with systemic vasoconstriction and cardiac stimulation

- Cerebral infarction (stroke)
- Myocardial infarction (heart attack)
- Ischaemic bowel (lack of blood flow to the gut resulting in tissue damage)
- Subarachnoid haemorrhage (bleeding in the protective covering of the brain)
- Various abnormal cardiac rhythms and asystole (lack of measurable cardiac activity)

Complications associated with CNS effects and muscles

- Fungal cerebritis (chronic use)
- Hyperprolactinaemia (high levels of prolactin leading to sexual dysfunction)
- Hyperthermia (raised temperature due to abnormal muscle and hypothalamic activity)
- Rhabdomyolysis (acute muscle breakdown leading to possible kidney damage by accumulation of the muscle breakdown product myoglobin)
- Seizures (occurring independently or in association with hyperthermia)

Chronic stimulant users often have a reduced libido and sexual performance with male impotence and female anorgasmia being common features. Amphetamine may also have a direct toxic effect on the kidneys. Some users have reported tooth and bone pain. Dry mouth and poor dental hygeine may explain the former but the reason for bone pain is unclear. Hyperactive children receiving methylphenidate chronically, have been reported as demonstrating reduced stature.

Treatment of acute CNS stimulant intoxication

The following information on acute CNS stimulant intoxication is for reference only. All cases of acute substance intoxication require referral to a National Poison Information Centre for current management advice.

General management

- Contact a Poisons Centre for current advice
- Hospitalisation is necessary
- Take appropriate action to empty the stomach in cases of oral stimulant ingestion (stimulants induce delayed gastric emptying times)
- Keep the patient in a quiet environment
- Recovery may take several days. Carers need to take precautions against patients attempting suicide

In most cases no specific measures are needed and patients recover uneventfully. However, in severe intoxication or in predisposed individuals medical problems will need specific management.

Anxiety and agitation[30,32,33]

Benzodiazepines are most often used to treat CNS stimulant induced anxiety and agitation with diazepam and chlordiazepoxide frequently being used. Doses are generally higher than those recommended for simple anxiety and benzodiazepines may need to be given for between one and three days. Typical regimens are as follows:

- Diazepam 5–10mg orally every four hours as tolerated.
- Chlordiazepoxide 25–50mg every four to six hours as

tolerated[28].

Hypertensive crisis

Acute CNS stimulant intoxication may be accompanied by dangerously raised blood pressure which may result in end organ damage to the kidneys and retina, and may predispose to cardiovascular complications such as heart attacks and strokes. Agents such as diazoxide, hydralazine, nitroprusside and phentolamine are currently indicated for use in such circumstances. Sublingual nifedipine has also been used[34].

Tachyarrhythmias (abnormal rapid cardiac rhythms)

Tachycardia with adequate cardiac output is probably best left untreated[30]. However life threatening arrhythmias may need to be treated with propranolol[28].

Unopposed alpha-adrenergic stimulation in the face of beta blockade has resulted in paradoxical hypertension. Appropriate antihypertensive cover is needed in such circumstances[28].

Ventricular arrhythmias in convulsive patients are best treated with disopyramide rather than lignocaine or mexiletine as the latter two may worsen seizures[30].

Psychotic episodes

Psychotic behaviour (often paranoid in nature) and hallucinations should be treated with neuroleptics. There is a wide variety of choice and much depends upon the clinician's preferences. Violently psychotic behaviour may be successfully managed with short acting neuroleptic depot preparations and conventional parenteral preparations when the oral route is not practicable. The use of the mental health act is appropriate in the treatment of such psychoses where there is a risk of self harm or injury to others or where the health of the patient is at risk.

Hyperthermia[32,33]

Hyperthermia may be due to a combination of lost hypothalamic control, and increased muscular activity. It has been identified as a significant mortality risk factor in CNS stimulant intoxication and may lead to rhabdomyolysis. It is treated with cold compresses, use of tepid sponging in combination with fanning or immersion in cool water.

There may also be a role for muscle relaxants, such as dantrolene.

Raised intracranial pressure

Several agents have been used in the treatment of raised intracranial pressure including hypertonic solutions of glucose, urea, mannitol, and glycerol. Dexamethasone and frusemide have also been used[35]. Hypertonic solutions set up a concentration gradient between the CNS and blood, drawing water from the intracranial areas while frusemide initiates a potent diuresis.

Seizures[32,33]

Seizures may occur independently or secondary to hyperthermia. Rectally or intravenously administered diazepam is used to control them.

Metabolic acidosis and electrolyte disturbances[30,32,33]

Metabolic acidosis may develop in severe intoxication. Although IV sodium bicarbonate administration is often used it may aggravate preexisting hypokalaemia and decrease the seizure threshold. Hypokalaemia is caused by stimulant induced shift of potassium from the blood into muscle tissue. It is treated with propranolol and may also require parenteral potassium administration.

Acid diuresis

Acid diuresis speeds the excretion of alkaline substances eg. amphetamine, by increasing their water solubility and subsequent renal tubular excretion. 2–4g of ascorbic acid in divided doses should be sufficient to accelerate amphetamine excretion.

CNS stimulant withdrawal syndrome

Stimulant use can rapidly result in dependence with a characteristic withdrawal syndrome. The speed at which dependence develops may correlate with the stimulants potency and method of administration. Rapid onset and high activity are thought to be risk factors for becoming dependent. Cocaine base

(Crack) is therefore particularly hazardous as it is inhaled as a vapour, and has the quickest onset of action.

Chronic stimulant use may lead to what is widely considered to be a psychological dependence. However some researchers believe that the characteristic after-depression, hypersomnolence (excessive sleeping) and hyperphagia (excessive eating) constitute a true withdrawal syndrome manifested predominantly psychologically. Regardless of this, the stimulant user eventually begins to experience an intense depression ('crash' or 'back ender') following periods of stimulant-induced euphoria.

It is this crash with subsequent stimulant craving coupled with continued tachyphylaxis that leads to daily or 'binge' stimulant use[27].

Acute withdrawal syndrome ('The Crash')

At the end of a binge episode, the stimulant user experiences extreme exhaustion and depression which last several hours. After this they crave sleep and may use benzodiazepines, alcohol, opioids or other sedative agents to alleviate their agitation and anxiety and allow them to sleep. This sleep is excessive. The individual wakes periodically to eat excessively (hyperphagia). This behaviour is termed the 'crash' and is symptomatic of stimulant withdrawal.

Chronic stimulant withdrawal syndrome

After the depression and hypersomnolence of the crash there usually follows an abstinence period from stimulants. The user's mood stabilises but they exhibit a lack of energy (anergia), general lack of interest in their surroundings and an inability to experience pleasure (anhedonia). Such feelings are intermittant, increasing over a period of up to a week or so after the crash. The user also experiences vivid memories of the drug-induced euphoria which are said to be 'persecuting' and cause intense psychological craving. Drug craving, anhedonia and anergia typically lead to the next binge episode.

The 'binge' cycle may be broken at this stage and if

abstinence is maintained for 6–18 weeks, the anhedonia and anergia slowly fade[27,28].

Therapies used to treat CNS stimulant withdrawal

Acute detoxification or 'crashing' from CNS stimulants usually requires no more than supervised support by appropriately trained professionals.

Depression, hypersomnolence and hyperphagia give way to intermittent anergia and anhedonia and drug craving over a period of days. The client may return to CNS stimulant use quickly after detoxification, and it is often not effective in maintaining prolonged CNS stimulant abstinence.

Psychotherapeutic treatment may be necessary to maintain abstinence and prevent relapse. Many different programmes are in existence taking various approaches. However, several phases are recognised in this treatment.

Firstly the aim is to break the 'binge' cycle, usually employing psychotherapy interventions. Prevention of relapse involves several steps including a period of enforced isolation from 'cues' to drug craving, (objects, situations, or people strongly associated with CNS stimulant use). Stimuli and cues are then reintroduced under controlled conditions, followed by the client reentering normal daily life where stimuli and cues are abundant. The client is then ideally supported in the community but often in practice is not[27].

Several drug regimens have been investigated as aids to CNS stimulant withdrawal management. All of these regimens require further rigorous clinical evaluation to assess their true benefit. The following information is taken from current reviews on the subject of stimulant (particularly cocaine) abuse and treatment[32,33].

Tricyclic antidepressants[33]

Most open trials with antidepressants have shown them to reduce stimulant craving and prolong abstinence. Agents investigated include imipramine (150–250mg daily), maprotiline (150mg daily), desipramine (100–200mg daily) and trazodone. Although further investigation is warranted, antidepressant therapy may be appropriate for several weeks to months. Whether all antidepressants show reduced stimulant craving also requires further investigation.

As tricyclic antidepressants take two to three weeks to work, they are of little help during the crash period but should be started early.

Current suggestions as to why tricyclic antidepressants should be useful suggest that they reverse the neurotransmitter receptor supersensitivity associated with chronic stimulant use. It is this receptor supersensitivity that is thought to cause both the depression and craving symptoms of withdrawal.

Carbamazepine[33,36]

Carbamazepine is an anticonvulsant with a tricyclic structure similar to the antidepressants. It is thought to reduce cocaine craving by reducing dopamine receptor supersensitivity. Typical 'study' doses ranged from 400–600mg daily. Clients were reported to tailor their doses to 200–400mg daily in one study.

Monoamine oxidase inhibitors (MAOI)[27,32,33,37]

MAOIs have been investigated in two US trials. Phenelzine was reported to be more effective and quicker acting against post-crash symptoms than tricyclics. They can also be used to discourage stimulant use. Concurrent use of MAOIs and stimulants can lead to a potentially fatal hypertensive interaction. The effects of MAOIs also is evident up to two weeks after discontinuation. Obviously, careful supervision and informed consent is necessary as the outcome of concurrent use can be disastrous[38].

Neurotransmitter precursors[33]

Neurotransmitter precursors are substances often present in the diet and used by the body in the synthesis of neurotransmitters. Neurotransmitter depletion occurs with chronic CNS stimulant use and has been suggested as one mechanism behind CNS stimulant withdrawal. However, such theories have not been supported in preclinical studies. Despite this, dietary neurotransmitter precursors such as tyrosine and tryptophan have been investigated in conjunction with tricyclics and bromocriptine. Although such combinations reduced subjective drug craving it is difficult to determine the neurotransmitter precursor contribution to this effect. Their efficacy requires further evaluation.

Dopamine agonists and stimulants[32,33]

Bromocriptine is reportedly faster in onset than tricyclic antidepressants in treating stimulant withdrawal and may be more useful for early crash symptoms. Bromocriptine/desipramine combinations are reported to be effective but require further investigation. Although long term bromocriptine efficacy or optimal dosage has not been established a suggested bromocriptine withdrawal regimen is as follows:

Day	Bromocriptine dose mg	Frequency
1–2	1.25	BD
3–4	1.25	TDS
5–6	2.5	BD
7–11	2.5	TDS
12–14	5	BD
15–20	Decrease by 50% every two days	

The stimulant methylphenidate has been investigated as a maintenance euphoric in cocaine users but has been reported to evoke intense euphoric memories and stimulant craving [4,33]. Maintenance amphetamines have been prescribed, sometimes in conjunction with heroin impregnated cigarettes[20].

Mazindol has been investigated by Berger *et al* and was reported to be dysphoric and 'free from abuse potential'. Mazindol reduced craving on the first day of administration (1–3mg mazindol daily) with reduced euphoria in those concurrently using cocaine[39].

Antipsychotics[33]

Antipsychotics have successfully been used to treat acute CNS stimulant-induced psychotic episodes. Their use to aid stimulant withdrawal is not well documented and there have been reports of antipsychotic agents increasing cocaine craving and prolonging binges.

Lithium[33]

It is of interest that stimulant abusers have a high incidence of specific underlying psychiatric complications notably mood disorders and attention deficit disorders. Lithium may be particularly useful in such patients but not others.

Lithium has been reported to attenuate cocaine-induced euphoria but not when cocaine was parenterally administered. It has also been reported to reduce cocaine use when administered concurrently.

Buspirone

Buspirone is a relatively new non-benzodiazepine anxiolytic. It acts by enhancing dopaminergic and noradrenergic CNS activity and by suppressing serotonergic activity. It has been shown to significantly improve withdrawal symptoms in cocaine users.

In conclusion, the benefits of drug therapies in ameliorating withdrawal symptoms and encouraging stimulant abstenance are equivocal and require further investigation. Compulsive stimulant use can be expected to stop when the client is prevented from obtaining the desired substance either physically or pychologically.

While acute detoxification and any concurrent medical problems can be managed pharmacologically, post-crash withdrawal needs intense psychotherapeutic intervention and possibly pharmacological aid to maintain abstinence.

Chapter 3
MDMA ('Ecstasy')

MDMA is a member of a class of drugs known by a variety of names including hallucinogenic or psychedelic amphetamines or entactogens[40]. Chemically, it is similar to amphetamine and the naturally occurring hallucinogenic alkaloid, mescaline. Examples of common hallucinogenic amphetamines are given below:

Common hallucinogenic amphetamines	
MDMA	3,4-dimethylenedioxymethamphetamine
MDA	3,4-dimethylenedioxyamphetamine
(Mescaline)	3,4,5-trimethoxyphenethylamine
TMA	3,4,5-trimethoxyphenylisopropylamine
DOM	2,5-dimethoxy - 4 methylphenylisopropylamine

Hundreds of variants to these drugs have been synthesised. DOM is extremely potent with a 20mg dose exerting its effects for up to three days whilst TMA causes aggression and hostility with megalomaniacal thoughts[4]. The exact modes of action of these compounds remains unknown but involves, in part, causing the release of 5 hydroxytrypamine in the CNS and neurotransmitter reuptake blockade[41].

MDMA and MDA ('The Love Drug') are probably the best known of the hallucinogenic amphetamines. They were synthesised in the early part of the twentieth century. In the 1970s and early 1980s, they were investigated for psychotherapeutic benefit, but proved unconvincing in this respect[40,41].

Currently both are restricted substances in America and Britain with no recognised medical applications. Both are widely used recreationally in America. MDMA is associated in Britain with popular youth dance culture ie. the Rave Scene[40].

MDMA has several properties making it attractive to the user including a stimulant effect, heightened perception, visual imagery and enhanced empathy towards those around one[40,42].

It is usually taken orally as tablets or capsules, but is sometimes injected (especially by those taking other drugs by the IV route).

Characteristics of MDMA intoxication

Usual Effects of MDMA (50–100mg orally)[40,41,42,43]

Onset 20–60 minutes:

Stimulant-like euphoria (not always present)

Calmness

Reduced anger and hostility

Increased empathy

Heightened perception

Overall stimulation (for dancing)

The above are generally the attractive properties of MDMA.

Other effects include the following:

Transient nausea/rarely vomiting

Dilated pupils

Tight jaw muscles (offset by gum chewing)

Sweating

Dry mouth

Reduced appetite

Insomnia

Increased heart rate

Transient rise then fall in blood pressure

Anorgasmia

Inability to sustain an erection

Rarely, users complain of numbness or tingling, luminescence of objects, enhanced colour acuity, movement of stationary objects (floor), crying, nystagmus (involuntary eye movement), unco-ordination and blurred vision.

Effects of higher MDMA doses[42,43]

Higher doses lead to additional effects, but susceptible individuals may experience these at lower doses.

- Tachycardia/palpitation
- Increased body temperature
- Increased muscle tone
- Visual hallucinations
- Anxiety/panic attacks

Rarely, individuals suffer serious medical complications that have led to several deaths.

Residual effects of MDMA use[42,43]

- Exhaustion
- Fatigue
- Muscle pain
- Depression
- Numbness
- Flashbacks

Users may, rarely, experience anxiety, rage and psychosis[43].

Medical complications of MDMA use

Acute and prolonged use of MDMA has been associated with several medical complications some of which have proved fatal. These include acute and chronic psychosis, malignant hyperthermia, disseminated intravascular coagulation (DIC), cardiac death, renal failure and haemorrhage.

Psychosis
Toxic psychosis may be seen when high MDMA doses are used.

It can be successfully treated with neuroleptics but haloperidol resistant psychosis has been reported[42,44].

Chronic psychosis has been reported in individuals with acute, chronic and high dose MDMA use. Treatment with haloperidol was effective in one patient who gradually improved but relapsed months later despite drug abstinence. Another responded partially to sulpiride but remained a psychiatric inpatient for three months[45].

Bizarre behaviour, presumably part of an acute psychosis, resulted in one accidental death by electrocution[46].

Sudden cardiac death

Increased heart rate, palpitations and labile blood pressure have all occured with MDMA ingestion, and may predispose to cardiac problems. A man with a history of a cardiac arrhythmia died after ingesting MDMA[47].

Disseminated intravascular coagulation (DIC)[40,48]

This is a condition where the insoluble plasma protein fibrin forms spontaneously intravascularly. Fibrin-Platelet aggregates deposit in the microvasculature of the body's organs blocking the blood supply and causing tissue damage. This is particularly dangerous with respect to the kidneys and lungs. Acute renal failure and several deaths due to respiratory failure have been reported secondary to DIC. Other complications of MDMA include hyperthermia and rhabdomyolysis. Rhabdomyolysis, DIC and a possible direct nephrotoxic effect of MDMA (similar to that suggested for amphetamine[49] may all have contributed to one case of acute renal failure[48].

Hyperthermia may be exacerbated by prolonged dancing and resultant dehydration. Accompanying convulsions have been reported. Treatment should involve effective seizure control and cooling measures. Intravenous dantrolene may be necessary[50].

Jaundice has also been reported[50] and several studies suggest that MDMA causes irreversible serotonergic neuronal damage in the brains of certain animals. MDMA and MDA users have reported increased susceptibility to minor infections (coughs, colds, herpes and candida)[43,51].

Tolerance and dependence

Tolerance to MDMA does occur with some chronic users taking up to 10 tablets over the course of an evening. Users have also been reported indulging in runs taking three to four tablets nightly. Animal models have suggested that dependence occurs but no cases of human MDMA dependence have yet been reported[40].

Chapter 4
LYSERGIC ACID
DIETHYLAMIDE (LSD)

LSD is the abbreviation of the German nomenclature for Lysergic Acid Diethylamide. It was synthesised in 1938 as an ergot alkaloid derivative but its psychedelic properties were not discovered until 1943. LSD has no recognised medical use and the hallucinogenic or illusogenic properties reside in the D (–) LSD-25 isomer[52,53].

Although described as the most potent hallucinogenic compound known, the term hallucinogen is a misnomer. The effects of the drug are very variable in the above respect, but the terms illusogenic or psychedelic are more apt as LSD will consistently produce perceptual and mood disturbances, and marked thought process alterations.

The mechanism of action of LSD is undetermined but it is thought to act by inhibiting central 5-hydroxytryptamine and stimulating dopaminergic activity. This is partly upheld by the fact that LSD intoxication has been managed with varying degrees of success by serotonin precursors and neuroleptic medications. The serotonin reuptake inhibitor fluoxetine has been reported to combat some of the after effects of LSD.

Desired effects of LSD[52,53]

The desired properties are difficult to determine as the drug effects are so very variable. LSD is commonly substituted for MDMA when mixed with amphetamine. Use may be experimental and 'the thing to do' as the effects are reported to be bizarre. Users have reported euphoria, relaxation, increased empathy, a pleasant dreamlike state, grossly altered perceptions, feelings of 'truth' and 'meaning' (mind expanding), and feelings of great insight and omnipotence.

Presentations of LSD[53]

LSD may be obtained illicitly in a different number of forms including small tablets (microdots), gelatin sheets, impregnated sugar cubes or paper (blotter acid). In these forms it is taken orally in doses of 100–250mcg. It has rarely been reported to have been administered nasally, intravenously, subcutaneously and conjunctivally in a liquid form.

Characteristics of acute LSD intoxication[52,53,54]

Doses as low as 20–25mcg can elicit a psychedelic effect with minimal effects on other organ systems. However, at doses of 0.5–2mcg/kg body weight peripheral signs of the drug are seen in minutes. Such effects are antimuscarinic and sympathomimetic in nature and are as follows:

- Markedly dilated pupils
- Raised blood pressure
- Increased heart rate
- Slightly raised body temperature
- Piloerection
- Hyper-reflexia
- Muscle weakness
- Nausea (and vomiting)
- Diarrhoea

These may persist for many hours and may be accompanied in the early stages by feelings of inner tension (relieved by laughing or crying) and mild euphoria.

After 2 to 3 hours the psychedelic effects become apparent. These manifest in a variety of ways including labile mood and grossly altered perceptions including illusions and hallucinations.

Mood alterations

Mood can fluctuate rapidly with users experiencing euphoria, depression, anxiety, elation and dysphoria all in a short period of time. Although euphoria usually predominates, anxiety can develop into severe panic attacks (a bad trip). Such panic may be caused by delusional beliefs or disturbing illusions/hallucinations and has resulted in self-injurous behaviour and traumatic accidents.

Perceptual changes

Users may experience heightened awareness of sensory input with extreme distortions of reality. Such distortions may be temporal, auditory, visual, tactile and delusional. Much of this is recognised as being drug-induced but may lead to extreme panic.
Examples of reported perceptual changes are listed below:

- Altered passage of time (fast or slower)
  Rapid ageing of oneself or others
  Magnification and distortions of sounds (auditory hallucinations are rare compared to intrinsic psychosis)

- Bright lights/patterns/colours on surrounding objects
  Distorted visual input (seeing objects as being something else)
  Trailing (movements perceived as a series of images blending and superimposing on other images)

- Various sensory hallucinations.
  Vivid thought/memories (often disturbing)
  Feeling of oneness with the universe (religious/mystical experiences)

- Synethesia (blending or overflow of sensory modalities where users report seeing sound and hearing colours)

Psychotic symptoms associated with LSD use are very varied and can mimic paranoid states or psychotic depression. However, hallucinations may differ from amphetamine-induced psychosis in having less auditory and paranoid components.

After 4 to 5 hours, if a major panic episode has not occurred, users can experience a sense of magical detachment and control over the surroundings. Attention is directed inwards on their perceived clarity and portentous quality of thought. Users often report a sense of truth or meaning, which is often far more important than what is perceived to be true or meant.

The whole episode begins to fade after about 12 hours. Some users have reported the experience as lasting much longer. However, the user is left with insomnia and weakness often accompanied by less pronounced illusions. Recovery is usually complete.

Treatment of acute LSD intoxication[52,55]

At doses usually employed medical complications are rare. Cases of accidental massive overdose (a user mistaking LSD for cocaine and inhaling it) has resulted in exaggerated sympathomimetic effects, coma and respiratory arrest. Hyperthermia and coagulation problems have rarely been reported.

However, users may present to a medical practitioner with LSD induced anxiety, psychosis, traumatic injury or behavioural abnormalities while acutely intoxicated.

While most cases of intoxication are self-limiting and require nothing more than a quiet, calm environment with supportive, nonjudgemental 'talk-down', some panic-stricken or frankly hallucinating or delusional patients will require pharmacological intervention.

For current advice, a National Poison Centre should be consulted. Unless massively overdosed, gastric emptying is useless but oral administration of activated charcoal may bind LSD in the stomach. However, this has not been established.

Severe agitation, hallucinations and psychosis have been successfully managed with benzodiazepines and neuroleptics administered by various routes. Miller*et al* reported the successful use of intramuscular lorazepam and haloperidol at doses of 2mg half-hourly until a response was achieved. Haloperidol has been used at standard doses of 5–20mg orally or intramuscularly. Miller advocates the intramuscular route as administration via other routes is more difficult in the hallucinating/deluded patient.

Other medicines used include L-tryptophan, a 5-hydroxytryptamine precursor. It is no longer widely available due to its association with eosinophilia myalgic syndrome.

After effects and characteristics of chronic LSD use

Neurological symptoms

Chronic use has been reported to lead to ataxia, slurred speech, dizziness, visual after images, incoordination and tremor. Convulsions have rarely been reported but are likely to effect predisposed individuals.

Tolerance

Tolerance can develop over a period of a few days but is lost just as quickly. There is a degree of cross-tolerance between LSD and mescaline and psylocibin.

Dependence/withdrawal

There are no reports of dependence or withdrawal in association with LSD.

Flashbacks

Flashbacks are a return of hallucinations or illusions after the immediate drug effect has worn off. It has been reported as presenting as visual intrusions or recurring images but other sensory modalities may be involved.

Flashbacks can result in transient depersonalisation, disorientation and anxiety. Use of alcohol or cannabis may trigger these episodes as may fatigue and movement into a dark environment. Frequency of occurrence is high with 23% of users reporting daily flashbacks, 18% reporting 2 to 3 episodes monthly and 43% reporting one every month or so in one study[52].

Flashbacks have been reported years after the last exposure to LSD. There would appear to be no currently recognised way of treating flashbacks.

Psychiatric illness

Clinicians have reported schizophrenic and schizoaffective illnesses occasionally being precipitated by the use of LSD. The affected individuals may in some way be predisposed to such psychiatric illness.

Chapter 5
PHENCYCLIDINE AND KETAMINE

Phencyclidine and ketamine are anaesthetic agents. Phencyclidine (PCP) was synthesised in the mid 1920s and by the 1950s it was licensed. However due to unwanted perioperative effects such as involuntary movements, seizures and postoperative psychological adverse effects, it was withdrawn in 1963 but remained in veterinary use after that time[4,56].

Ketamine is chemically similar to PCP and was introduced in 1965. Although demonstrating similar psychological effects to PCP, it is less prone to cause seizures.

PCP is widely used recreationally in the USA, whereas ketamine is used both in the USA and the UK. Physical dependence has not yet been recognised although psychological dependence may occur.

There are similarities between the patterns of chronic use of stimulants and PCP including repeated drug administration ending in confusion, depression and sleep. However there are currently no pharmacological withdrawal or maintenance considerations for ketamine or PCP[57].

Because of their chemical and pharmacological similarities, it is expected that ketamine-associated complications be treated as those associated with PCP. Indeed, the signs and symptoms of ketamine and PCP intoxication are easily mistaken for one another[59,60].

The desired effects of ketamine and PCP

When used recreationally, it is often found that novice users dislike the drug-induced sensory isolation and will not go on to repeat the experience, however regular users state that it dissolves their anxieties and tensions[58].

Smoking PCP allows the user to titrate the dosage for desired effects. Other routes of administration i.e. oral, IV or snorting the drug, do not lend themselves to such titration and can lead to unpredictable effects[59]. Favoured effects of ketamine and PCP are listed below:

- Flying/floating sensations
- 'CNS stimulant-like' euphoria
- Perceptual and cognitive distortions of time, place and person
- Sensory distortions
- Numbness
- Incoordination
- Feelings of strength/power/invulnerability
- Hallucinations

Effects of chronic administration

Chronic PCP users indulge in 'runs' or repeated drug administrations for a few days without food or rest. The run ends with disorientation, depression and sleep. Whether this is a withdrawal syndrome is debatable. Tolerance has not been demonstrated although anecdotal tolerance has been reported with doses ranging from 5–10mg (smoked) to 80–100mg by other routes, taken two to three times daily. There have also been unconfirmed reports of PCP consumption up to 1g over a 24-hour period. Reported effects of chronic PCP use are as follows:

- Memory impairment
- 'Flash backs'
- Inarticulate speech, including stuttering
- Anxiety

- Depression
- Social withdrawal
- Isolation
- Unpredictable violent behaviour
- Toxic psychosis
- Mutism

Characteristic of acute PCP and ketamine intoxication[56,57,58]

As the dosage increases, all observed effects become magnified and others will become apparent.

Low dosage use

- Euphoria (stimulant-like)
- Sedation/apathy
- Stimulation
- Dissociation
- Floating/flying
- Distortions of space and time
- Sensory distortions
- Slurred speech
- Small pupils with blurred vision
- Dizziness
- Mutism
- Hostility/violence
- Confusion, terror
- Catatonic rigidity (PCP)
- Cataleptic rigidity (k)
- Sweating
- Hyperacousis (very sensitive hearing)

- Loss of response to pin-prick
- Nystagmus (horizontal/vertical)
- Echolalia (repeating what is said to one)

High dosage use
- Analgesia/anaesthesia
- Drowsiness/sleeping
- Prolonged coma (PCP)
- Hypertension
- Tachycardia
- Sweating
- Nausea/vomiting
- Hallucinations
- Nystagmus (involuntary eye movements)
- Double vision
- Increased salivation
- Convulsions (possibly status epilepticus)
- Involuntary muscle movements
- Acute toxic psychosis
- Hyperthermia (raised body temperature)
- Reduced corneal reflexes
- Skeletal muscle breakdown (rhabdomyolysis)
- Renal failure ($2°$ to rhabdomyolysis and hypotension)
- Increased shallow respiratory rate
- Labile blood pressure
- Postural spasm
- Death

Acute toxic psychosis
Both PCP and ketamine can produce an acute toxic psychosis consisting of hallucinations, delusions, disorganised thought,

distorted body image and dissociation. It has been reported to consist of three phases:

i) Several hours to days — the patient may be confused and paranoia may be present.

ii) 48 hours to several days — the patient will be agitated.

iii) Up to 2 weeks — the patient begins to normalise. (There have however been reported cases where this has taken up to a year with PCP)

Mortality

PCP-associated deaths commonly result from behavioural abnormalities including suicide, homicide and accidents[58]. Users have attempted to heighten dissociative effects by swimming. Death by drowning has resulted[56]. Death due to acute overdose (150–200mg) is rare but has resulted from status epilepticus, respiratory arrest, cardiovascular collapse or hyperpyrexia[56,58]. Ketamine associated deaths are rare but a similar potential exists as ketamine can cause abnormal behaviour.

Treatment of acute PCP intoxication

The following information on acute PCP intoxication is for reference only. All cases of acute substance intoxication require referral to a National Poisons Centre for current management advice.

General management

- Contact a Poisons Centre for current advice.
- Keep the patient in a quiet environment (this is often all that is needed).
- Severe toxicity and coma may necessitate the use of certain drug elimination enhancement techniques.

Acid diuresis[4,58]

As the majority of PCP is hepatically metabolised, this technique has been questioned. Myoglobinuria (myoglobin in the urine) is an absolute contraindication to acid diuresis.

Nasogastric suction[58]

Removal of gastric secretions enhances excretion.

Activated charcoal[4,58]

Oral administration of activated charcoal prevents absorption from the gastrointestinal tract regardless of the route of administration.

Seizures

Generalised tonic-clonic and rarely focal seizures can present at any stage of intoxication. They have been successfully treated with 5–10mg PR/IV diazepam, (up to 30mg). Refractory cases may require further investigations including blood glucose, core temperature, U+Es and acid-base balance.

Concomitant hyperthermia requires aggressive anti-seizure therapy and neuromuscular blockade may be required.

Some neuroleptics may precipitate seizures in predisposed individuals. Chlorpromazine and loxapine have been reported to be epileptogenic. Haloperidol and zuclopenthixol should be used with caution. Thioridazine and pimozide have the least potential for exacerbating seizures[61].

Psychosis

Haloperidol and chlorpromazine have been used successfully with cases of intoxication. (The psychosis may last for several days). Short-acting depot preparations may be of some use but consideration should be given to the seizure exacerbating effects of the neuroleptic employed.

Dystonic reactions

Localised dystonia involving the neck and tongue have been reported. Diphenhydramine (50mg IV) has successfully abated such reactions but is not available in the UK. Procyclidine 5mg

IV will usually control drug-induced dystonias within 5 minutes. Occasionally 10mg is necessary. The intramuscular route will delay the drug response but may be more convenient in the psychotic individual.

Urinary retention

High doses are associated with atropine-like effects notably urinary retention. Urinary catheterisation may be necessary.

Hypertension

There is a 50% incidence of related hypertension, usually only lasting for several hours amongst PCP and ketamine users. Such episodes are less severe when agitation is controlled. If hypertension continues then standard antihypertensive measures may be necessary.

Pyrexia

An increase in body temperature is usually moderate. It can occur more acutely in agitated or comatose individuals, in whom temperature monitoring is precautionary. Hyperthermia rarely occurs but should be treated with such cooling measures as ice baths or cooling blankets (etc). Malignant hyperthermia is treated with cooling measures and dantrolene is a treatment option.

Aggressive/violent behaviour

Benzodiazepines (PR/oral/IM diazepam) are recommended for such behaviour. Intramuscular neuroleptics e.g. haloperidol have also been used. Intramuscular chlorpromazine has been associated with sudden death of some patients. There has also been concern over administration of intramuscular neuroleptics to struggling patients and this has been suggested as a risk factor for sudden death.

Coma

Intoxicated patients may rapidly progress to coma; this can last from hours to days depending upon the drug dosage used. Rarely, apnoea and respiratory depression occur and is more prevalent in children. Complications can include aspiration pneumonia and rhabdomyolysis.

It is recommended that comatose, psychotic and catatonic patients have urine analysis for haematuria. The appearance of myoglobin will necessitate hospitalisation.

Chapter 6
CANNABIS

Cannabis is the term used for a group of compounds that occur in the plant material of cannabis sativa. In the UK, cannabis is legally regarded as any part of any plant of the genus cannabis[62].

Other names for cannabis are Marijuana and Hashish. It may present as leaf material, resin or liquid and contains several active ingredients.

Active ingredients of cannabis

- Delta 9-tetrahydrocannabinol (Dronabinol/delta 9-THC)
- Delta 8-tetrahydrocannabinol (delta 8-THC)
- Delta 9-tetrahydrocannabinolic acid

Desired effects of cannabis[63]

- Elation/euphoria
- Distortion of time and place
- Sedation
- Mental relaxation
- Acuity of sensation
- Silliness/gregariousness

These effects may last for one to three hours with the individual returning to normal without the 'hangover effect' associated with alcohol.

Other effects

Other effects of cannabis at 'normal' doses include the following[63,64,65]:

- Transient floating sensation
- Loss of concentration
- Tachycardia
- Mild sweating
- Bloodshot eyes
- Dry mouth
- Lowered blood pressure (on standing)
- Tremor/ataxia
- Nausea and/or vomiting
- Elevated blood pressure (supine)
- Hunger

As the dose is increased other effects maybecome apparent[60,61].

- Lethargy/irritability
- Disturbed memory/judgement/confusion
- Anxiety/paranoia
- Depersonalisation
- Panic/intense fear
- Depression
- Hallucination
- Psychotic episodes

Chronic cannabis use may cause gynaecomastia (breast development in males) disrupted fertility and reduced respiratory function (smoking). The amotivational syndrome has been reported in chronic users but there are still arguments as to whether this is caused by excessive use[64].

Dependence[64]

It is widely accepted that cannabis is not addictive and is safe to use. New evidence is accumulating both from animal and human studies which suggests otherwise. Some studies have demonstrated tolerance to cannabis with high doses and prolonged use. Withdrawal effects have been shown in both animal models and humans and is reported to have certain similarities to opioid withdrawal. Other studies have failed to demonstrate such a withdrawal syndrome.

Although findings are conflicting, cannabis cannot be assumed to be totally free from causing dependence in some users.

Treatment

The following is for reference only. All cases of acute substance intoxication require referral to a National Poisons Information Centre for current management advice. Psychological withdrawal symptoms have been managed when necessary with low doses of benzodiazepines.

Mild panic usually requires no treatment besides verbal reassurance and avoidance of stimulants (caffeine, amphetamines etc). More pronounced panic episodes may require the administration of benzodiazepines.

Acute psychotic/paranoid reactions rarely occur. They are often associated with perplexation and disorientation when large doses of cannabis are taken. Cannabis may also exacerbate schizophrenia in susceptible individuals. Neuroleptic drugs are used to manage such episodes.

Chapter 7
NON-OPIOID CENTRAL NERVOUS SYSTEM DEPRESSANTS

Non-opioid CNS depressants include the benzodiazepines, barbiturates and certain hypnotic (sleep inducing) agents. Medicinally such drugs are, or have been used to treat anxiety, insomnia, and epilepsy. Some benzodiazepines are also used as muscle relaxants especially in the orthopaedic setting.

These drugs generally produce progressive depression of the CNS characterised by sedation and sleep, sometimes preceded by a period of paradoxical excitement and disinhibition.

Dependence may develop with prolonged use. A withdrawal syndrome is well recognised with barbiturates and is more dangerous than opioid withdrawal. A benzodiazepine withdrawal syndrome is also recognised but is less well defined. Cross tolerance and cross dependence generally occurs between the above drugs

Barbiturates

The following is a list of available barbiturates:
- Amylobarbitone
- Butobarbitone
- Quinalbarbitone
- Phenobarbitone
- Pentobarbitone
- Hexobarbitone

- Thiopentone

These agents are now, with the exception of phenobarbitone, rarely used, and barbiturate use has declined dramatically due to changes in their legal classification and their displacement by the benzodiazepines as hypnotic or sedative agents.

Characteristics of Acute Barbiturate Intoxication[66]

- Slurred speech
- Inattentiveness
- Drunken behaviour
- Ataxia (progressing with intoxication)
- Nystagmus (progressing with intoxication)
- Drowsiness
- Sleep
- Coma
- Respiratory depression
- Cheyne - Stoke respiration
- Apnoea
- Respiratory arrest
- Tachycardia
- Hypotension
- Cyanosis
- Shock
- Death

Other complications may include hypothermia (rarely fever), congestive heart failure, cardiac arrhythmias, pulmonary oedema, pneumonia and renal failure. Skin blisters occurring between the fingers and backs of knees are common.

Treatment of Acute Barbiturate Intoxication[67, 68]

The following information on acute barbiturate intoxication is for reference only. All cases of acute substance intoxication require referral to a National Poisons Information Centre for current management advice.

General Management

Barbiturate overdose carries a high mortality rate reported at between 3 and 6% overall and as high as 32% in severe coma. Treatment is largely supportive consisting of adequate airways maintenance and assisted respiration where necessary. Gastric lavage with ipecacuanha mixture is recommended within four hours of ingestion, whilst repeated oral doses of activated charcoal enhance elimination. Usual doses are 50g four hourly or 25g two hourly.

Phenobarbitone elimination may be enhanced by forced alkaline diuresis with sodium bicarbonate. The severely poisoned patient will require haemodialysis or haemoperfusion to remove the drug. Hypotension may be combated with plasma volume expanders whilst difficult cases have required dopamine or dobutamine where preservation of renal blood flow was critical.

Characteristics of Barbiturate Withdrawal[66, 69, 70]

Chronic barbiturate administration followed by abrupt discontinuation may result in a severe withdrawal syndrome similar to that seen in alcoholics. Onset of withdrawal depends on the duration of action of the barbiturate used and usually occurs after 8 to 12 hours of abstinence from the shorter acting agents. Phenobarbitone persists in the body for several days and abrupt discontinuation may result in a mild withdrawal syndrome with a prolonged time to onset. The following is a list of signs and symptoms associated with barbiturate withdrawal syndrome:

- Anorexia/nausea and vomiting/abdominal cramps
- Distorted perception/delirium
- Psychosis with visual/auditory hallucinations (may be delayed)
- Convulsions (16 hrs to 5 days after the last dose)
- Restlessness/anxiety/irritability
- Coarse tremor

- Increased muscle tone
- Brisker deep tendon reflexes
- Ankle clonus
- Fasciculation or twitching
- Insomnia
- Sweating
- Hypotension
- Rapid sitting pulse (100/min) increasing by 15/min on standing

Treatment of barbiturate withdrawal syndrome

A withdrawal syndrome can occur within 8 to 12 hours of abstinence from short acting barbiturates and may be mild or severe. Treatment consists of administration of a stabilising dose of barbiturate to suppress withdrawal. Even severely dependent patients can usually be successfully withdrawn from barbiturates in two to three weeks.

Teggin and Bewley[66] reported a successful withdrawal protocol by first substituting the client's barbiturates for 1000mg of short acting pentobarbitone given daily in four divided doses. The initial stabilising dose was reduced in the face of impending intoxication and increased appropriately if withdrawal symptoms persisted. This stabilising dose was then maintained for three days being reduced by 100mg per day thereafter until complete withdrawal was achieved. Patients were observed for another 48 hours after this time.

Alternatively, the long-acting barbiturate, pheno-barbitone has been added as the stabilising barbiturate. Initially the clients' total daily barbiturate intake is ascertained and replaced by 30mg phenobarbitone for each 100–200mg short acting barbiturate used. If the client demonstrates a withdrawal syndrome on the first day a single 100–200mg phenobarbitone dose may be administered. After an appropriate stabilising dose has been established the total daily dose may be decreased by 30mg each day, until the drug has been completely discontinued (see also 'illicit drug use in pregnancy').

Benzodiazepines

Since the introduction of the first benzodiazepine, chlordiazepoxide, in 1960 well over 500 million people have been exposed to this class of drug[71]. Initially benzodiazepines were marketed as being free of dependence potential but cases of dependence and withdrawal were increasingly reported during the early 1980s. Currently, various benzodiazepines are used for short-term management of anxiety states, sleep disturbances and forms of epilepsy. They are also used as pre-operative medications, short-term muscle relaxants and in alcohol and drug detoxification. Because of their now widely recognised dependence potential, their use in anxiety treatment is diminishing but their role as hypnotics remains with an estimated million chronic users currently present in Britain.

Mechanism of action

Benzodiazepines exert their effects by reducing CNS neuronal activity. They have been found to have a specific receptor in the CNS (particularly in an area of the brain called the limbic system). Currently it is thought that benzodiazepines bind to the benzodiazepine receptors and potentiate the effects of the inhibitory neurotransmitter, Gamma-aminobutyric acid (GABA)[72]. It is GABA that ultimately reduces electrical CNS activity by stabilising neuronal cell membranes. Benzodiazepines also alter noradrenaline and 5-hydroxytryptamine metabolism[71].

Barbiturates also potentiate GABA activity but not through specific receptors, whilst chlormethiazole is thought to act via GABA-A receptors.

Consequences of long-term use

Many patients take benzodiazepines regularly without reporting any adverse effects. However long term use can lead to the following[73]:

- Memory impairment (improves on discontinuation)
- Tiredness
- Drowsiness/lassitude
- Psychomotor slowing
- Ataxia
- Confusion

Paradoxical responses occur in up to 5% of benzodiazepine users. These may be as follows:

- Aggression/excitement
- Hostility
- Sexual impropriety
- Labile emotional responses

Patients may crave benzodiazepines between doses especially with very short-acting agents such as alprazolam and lorazepam. This is the beginning of a withdrawal syndrome despite continued use and is attributed to drug tolerance[74].

List of benzodiazepines		
	Hypnotics	**Anxiolytics**
Short-acting:	Loprazolam	Alprazolam
	Lormetazolam	Bromazepam
	Temazepam	Lorazepam
		Oxazepam
Longer-acting	Flunitrazepam	Chlordiazepoxide
	Flurazepam	Clobazam
	Nitrazepam	Clorazepate
		Diazepam
		Midazolam

All benzodiazepines work in much the same way and the distinction between hypnotics and anxiolytics is more a function of commercial marketing strategy than any differences in pharmacology.

Characteristics of acute benzodiazepine intoxication[75,76]

- Drowsiness
- Ataxia
- Unconsciousness
- Confusion/slurred speech
- Coma
- Diminished reflexes
- Hypotension
- Seizures
- Respiratory depression
- Apnoea

Treatment of acute benzodiazepine intoxication

The following information on acute benzodiazepine intoxication is for reference only. All cases of acute substance intoxication require referral to a National Poisons Information Centre for current management advice.

General management

Benzodiazepine intoxication alone is rarely fatal. Coma, seizures and cardiac arrest are rare and seen more often when benzodiazepines are combined with alcohol or other CNS depressants. Treatment is largely supportive.

Recent benzodiazepine ingestion should be managed by ipecacuanha emesis in conscious patients and gastric lavage in the unconscious patient. Activated charcoal may also be used after emesis or gastric lavage.

Hypotension is controlled with intravenous fluid administration and pressor agents where necessary.

Drug Treatment

Currently, no drug is licensed in the UK specifically to treat benzodiazepine overdose. However flumazenil is a benzodiazepine antagonist licensed for the reversal of sedation due to benzodiazepines in anaesthesia, the intensive care setting and for diagnostic procedures. It is administered as a 200mcg slow intravenous bolus followed by 100mcg every minute to 1mg (2mg in the intensive care setting)[77]. Despite being unlicensed, the drug has been used to reverse intoxication in cases of benzodiazepine overdose. Concern has been expressed over its use in dependent individuals as it may precipitate a full withdrawal syndrome. There have also been reports of deaths associated with flumazenil administration in cases of multiple drug intoxication (e.g. benzodiazepines and tricyclic antidepressants)[78,79].

Benzodiazepine dependence

Estimates of the incidence of benzodiazepine dependence vary greatly. Quotes vary from 15–44%[80], less than a third of benzodiazepine users[81] and up to 100%[82,83]. This variation in incidence may reflect the defining criteria used for diagnosing dependence. The figure of about a third is widely used, but the majority of chronic benzodiazepine users will experience withdrawal symptoms of some form, however mild, on discontinuation of their medication[74].

Tyrer[80] and Ashton[74] have suggested certain factors as predisposing to benzodiazepine dependence. These include:

- High benzodiazepine doses for prolonged periods
- Premorbid personality
- Borderline personality disorders
- Dependent and avoidant personality

It would appear that because benzodiazepines work best in individuals who are anxious, these people self-select for chronic administration. Vulnerable, anxious people with poor ability to cope with stress are more likely to continue using benzodiazepines[74]. Joughin found that a history of depression was associated with poorer chance of successful benzodiazepine discontinuation than patients suffering anxiety alone[84].

Dependence and withdrawal symptoms can occur after only four to six weeks of treatment[80]. Finley and Nolan reported benzodiazepine withdrawal in a ventilated patient following discontinuation of midazolam after 21 days of treatment[81].

Benzodiazepine withdrawal syndrome

Benzodiazepine withdrawal syndrome usually begins a few days after stopping the medication. For shorter-acting benzodiazepines this will be 2 to 3 days[70] although some patients demonstrate withdrawal between doses of very short-acting benzodiazepines without discontinuing their medication[74]. Discontinuation of longer-acting benzodiazepines such as diazepam leads to withdrawal symptoms in 7 to 10 days[73].

In most cases, the symptoms are prevalent for between one to six weeks. However some symptoms may persist in a small set of clients for several months and this has been termed chronic or post-withdrawal syndrome[73]. The explanation for benzodiazepine dependence and withdrawal focuses on changing benzodiazepine receptor numbers. Overstimulation of the receptors is proposed to cause their down regulation (decreased numbers). Benzodiazepine discontinuation or tolerance leads to reduced inhibitory transmitter (GABA) activity with the emergence of the withdrawal syndrome[74].

Characteristics of the benzodiazepine withdrawal syndrome

Withdrawal syndrome is precipitated within days of stopping benzodiazepines and in some cases may persist for many months. Patients may report the following[73,76,86]:

- Anxiety/apprehension/unease/insomnia/tremor
- Palpitations
- Dizziness/unsteadiness
- Agoraphobia/panic attacks
- Muscle twitching/jerking/spasms/pain
- Poor concentration/memory
- Depersonalisation/feeling of unreality
- Heightened perception

- Numbness of extremities
- Burning sensations or creeping of the skin
- Objects appearing to move
- Weakness in the neck/head/jaw/limbs
- Blurred vision/sore eyes
- Toothache/headache
- Nausea and vomiting/diarrhoea or constipation/dysphagia/abdominal pain
- Influenza-like syndrome/malaise
- Breast/mammary pain
- Menorrhagia
- Loss/increased appetite
- Thirst/polyuria
- Urinary incontinence (rarely)
- Acute psychotic episodes
- Hallucinations
- Seizures

Depersonalisation and feelings of unreality coupled with waxing and waning perceptual distortions are very disturbing. Patients may think they are 'going mad'. Toothache has resulted in unnecessary extractions whilst blurred vision has prompted patients to visit their optician. The flu-like syndrome often starts within a few weeks of stopping benzodiazepines and lasts a month or longer. Seizures are associated with abrupt discontinuation of short-acting benzodiazepines in particular. Vivid memories and nightmares may also prove troublesome.

Management of benzodiazepine discontinuation and the withdrawal syndrome

It is often the patient who initiates steps to discontinue benzodiazepines, being prompted from several corners including media pressure, a history of adverse events on benzodiazepines and encouragement or pressure from family, friends and doctor[73].

Without the patient's full, informed co-operation successful discontinuation is unlikely. The process of benzodiazepine discontinuation is usually undertaken in an outpatient setting[73,80]. The inpatient setting is currently regarded as suitable only for those clients who have experienced particularly severe withdrawal symptoms (ie. psychosis, fits) on previously unsuccessful attempts[80,86].

Preparing to discontinue a client's benzodiazepines involves a number of steps including consideration of medical and drug histories, maintaining client confidence in the process and assessing the client's worries, expectations and sources of support. Clients and their families should always be appropriately informed. Anxiety management programmes and relaxation programmes may be of use as withdrawal is begun.

Certain clients may be deemed unsuitable for benzodiazepine withdrawal, chronic epileptics using benzodiazepines for seizure control being an example. Elderly clients who are maintained on low doses symptom-free and those being successfully treated for chronic/severe anxiety or insomnia are other examples[87].

Benzodiazepine discontinuation in the chronic user is done gradually over a relatively long period of time. Many benzodiazepines are not available in a suitable range of strengths to allow small dosage reductions. Diazepam is available in a range of tablet strengths and syrups. Patients are commonly transferred to an equivalent dose of diazepam prior to discontinuation. Whilst this will avoid breakthrough withdrawal symptoms associated with shorter-acting benzodiazepines, day time drowsiness may be problematic.

Diazepam substitution

It is important to note that anxiolytic equivalence and substitution equivalence are not the same. Whilst 1mg of lorazepam is equivalent to 5mg of diazepam in anxiolytic terms it is equivalent to 10mg of diazepam when substituting so as to avoid withdrawal symptoms. The following table provides a guide to benzodiazepine equivalence for the purposes of substitution.

Once the client's reported daily benzodiazepine intake has been estimated in terms of milligrams of diazepam the substitution process can begin. It usually takes about a week but should be tailored to the patient's needs.

Table of benzodiazepine substitution equivalence[80,86,88,89]			
Drug	Half-life (active metabolite) (hours)		Dose equivalent to 10mg diazepam
Alprazolam	6–20		1
Bromazepam	9–20		6
Chlordiazepoxide	5–30	(36–200)	20–25
Clobazam	9–60		20
Clorazepate		(36–200)	15
Diazepam	21–46	(36–200)	<u>10</u>
Flunitrazepam	35	(200)	1
Flurazepam	47–95	(40–250)	15–30
Loprazolam	7–20		1–2
Lorazepam	8–25		1–2
Lormetazepam	10–12		1–2
Midazepam	1–7	(36–200)	10
Nitrazepam	15–38		20 (10–40)
Oxazepam	4–15		40 (30–80)
Temazepam	5–22		20
(This table is only to be used as a guide to initial substitution doses of diazepam. Individuals may require adjustment so as to avoid withdrawal symptoms).			

The clients' benzodiazepine regimen is recommended to be substituted gradually in one dose stages. It is best illustrated by example:

- If a client is taking lorazepam 2mg three times daily, substitution should begin by replacing the last daily dose with diazepam (20mg). Two days later the midday

dose should be substituted and finally two days after
that the morning dose. On the fourth day after the
initial evening substitution, the client would be
receiving a total daily dose of 60mg diazepam.

It has been argued that the initial 'last daily dose' substitution is
questionable as it may lead to sleep disturbances with consequent
loss of patient confidence. Some practitioners therefore start by
substituting the midday dose.

Some patients feel better having short-acting benzodiazepines replaced in this way and possibly avoiding breakthrough withdrawal between doses. Others apparently have great
difficulty substituting in this manner and the substitution may
need to be more gradual[86,89]

Diazepam discontinuation

Higgitt *et al* reported a successful technique whereby the rate of
dosage reduction was titrated against withdrawal symptoms[80].
Dose decrements (0.5 to 2.5mg) were made at weekly intervals
until withdrawal symptoms became apparent. The rate of
reduction was then reduced and guided by the patient's
willingness to proceed further. This process was continued to the
last few milligrams of diazepam. Placebo or alternate day dosing
was employed to finally attain complete discontinuation.

Some practitioners have adopted the arbitrary principle of
one month of reduction per year of benzodiazepine use. This may
result in withdrawal regimens of between 6 months and two years
duration. Such protracted regimens are associated with poor
outcome[73].

Lader and Morton aimed to withdraw clients in six weeks
and in up to twelve weeks in difficult cases. The rate of withdrawal
was tailored to that which the patient could tolerate. Patients could
manage large dose decrements initially but required small
reductions in dosage as the withdrawal process progressed.
Proportional dose decrements rather than absolute ones were
considered more appropriate[73].

Joughin *et al* investigated an inpatient benzodiazepine

withdrawal regimen over four weeks. It was heavily supported in a group setting with benzodiazepines being withdrawn in eight equal decrements over the month. Despite the support a six month follow up showed only 38% successful withdrawal. Poor outcome in terms of successful withdrawal was associated with a pre-existing history of depression[84].

Taylor published guidelines for benzodiazepine withdrawal for Dulwich Hospital, London[89]. Recommendations included decreasing diazepam doses at weekly, fortnightly or monthly intervals as tolerated by the patient. The size of dosage reductions were determined by the daily diazepam dose and are outlined as follows:

Daily diazepam dose	Decrement
>15–20mg	2mg
10–15mg	1mg
5mg	0.5mg

Such a regimen would allow a client to withdraw from 30mg of diazepam in just over 6 months assuming that only weekly decrements were employed.

A benzodiazepine withdrawal protocol is contained in the British National Formulary[90.] It suggests a transfer to diazepam and fortnightly decrements of 2 to 2.5mg until withdrawal symptoms emerge. The situation is to be maintained until symptoms improve and withdrawal continued in smaller fortnightly decrements in the above fashion until complete discontinuation.

The general rule for all benzodiazepine withdrawal regimens is to decrease the dose as quickly and comfortably as the **client** wishes to go. The process may take as little as six weeks or as long as several months.

Adjunctive medications used during benzodiazepine withdrawal
Several drugs have been used in attempts to alleviate benzodiazepine withdrawal symptoms. There have been reports

of partial success with some of these and contradicting claims have been made for others. Currently there is no 'magic cure' with no drug specifically licensed for withdrawal management.

Antidepressants: Antidepressants are advocated if there is a co-existing or emerging depression[90]. It has been suggested that they are more useful in the later phases of withdrawal and that their sedative effects may combat insomnia. Imipramine and clomipramine may be effective for panic and phobic symptoms.

Their gradual introduction may be more acceptable to the client and they may need to be maintained for several months[73]. Antidepressants should also be withdrawn gradually[90]. However tricyclic antidepressants are toxic in overdose, and Joughin *et al* encountered two suicides in the 21 client study group[84]. The 5-hydroxytryptamine reuptake inhibitors antidepressants (fluvoxamine, fluoxetine, paroxetine, sertraline) are safer in this respect. However, most antidepressants can exacerbate seizures which are one of the features of early benzodiazepine withdrawal syndrome.

Anticonvulsants: Several anticonvulsants have been investigated as adjuvants during benzodiazepine discontinuation. Carbamazepine has been reported to reduce the incidence of withdrawal seizures and the severity of the withdrawal syndrome at doses up to 800mg daily[91].

Phenytoin, sodium valproate and clonazepam have all been successfully used to combat withdrawal seizures. Valproate and clonazepam (a benzodiazepine) have both been reported to reduce the severity of other withdrawal symptoms[93].

Clonidine: Clonidine is widely used to alleviate opioid withdrawal symptoms. Reports of its efficacy in benzodiazepine withdrawal are mixed, but moderate success has been reported[92].

Propranolol: Propranolol may be useful to alleviate some of the physical signs of anxiety such as tremor, muscle twitching, palpitations and sweating[89], but the BNF advises its use only when other approaches have failed[90].

Neuroleptics (antipsychotics): Neuroleptics may be required to manage hallucinations or psychosis. However, they may worsen withdrawal symptoms or precipitate seizures[80,90]. Low anxiolytic neuroleptic doses are not useful[73] and emergence of severe withdrawal symptoms (hallucinations, psychosis, seizures) indicates that benzodiazepines are being discontinued too rapidly.

Flumazenil: Flumazenil is a benzodiazepine antagonist used to treat benzodiazepine intoxication in certain clinical settings. However, it may also have a role in alleviating withdrawal symptoms[77]. It is of interest that flumazenil has reversed benzodiazepine tolerance in epileptic patients without inducing withdrawal fits[94].

Lader and Morton reported the use of flumazenil in abstinent clients complaining of withdrawal symptoms. Intravenous administration (up to 2mg in divided doses) reduced symptoms for up to 24 hours in some patients[73] but further investigation into the efficacy and safety of this promising agent is required.

Illicit intravenous benzodiazepine use

The problem of illicit intravenous use is entirely separate from that posed by long-term oral administration of prescribed benzodiazepines. It is a practice that has been growing since the 1980s in the UK and those involved have also been identified as being involved in other illicit drug use.

Temazepam has lent itself particularly to this activity due to its formulation as a liquid or gel filled capsule. Its growing popularity is illustrated by the marked increase in demand for illicit temazepam capsules in Glasgow in 1987. The 'street' price increased from 20 pence to £2.50 per capsule[95]. Such practises are not without risk and apart from the potential for spreading blood borne diseases via needle sharing, other immediate problems have been reported.

Intra-arterial administration of the content of gel-filled capsules has resulted in venous thrombosis, tissue ischaemia and muscle breakdown. Treatment of such conditions has involved heparinisation, forced alkaline diuresis (to avoid renal failure secondary to muscle breakdown) and surgical intervention. Despite intensive therapy some patients have undergone amputation of the affected limbs[96,97]. There have been calls to discontinue gel-filled capsules[98,99], and many health authorities and general practitioners have begun using temazepam tablets to help combat the problem of injecting. However, while reporting a higher incidence of deep vein thrombosis with gel-filled rather than liquid-filled capsules, Fox *et al* also noted that temazepam tablets have been dissolved and injected[100].

Chlormethiazole

Chlormethiazole was introduced in 1957, a few years after thalidomide and before chlordiazepoxide. It is a chemical derivative of thiamine and is currently licensed for the short-term treatment of insomnia, restlessness, agitation in the elderly and hospital-supervised alcohol detoxification. When administered parenterally, it is used to treat pre-eclamptic toxaemia, eclampsia, status epilepticus and as a sedative during regional anaesthesia. While being relatively safe at prescribed doses, prolonged use can lead to tolerance and dosage escalation with some rare individuals taking up to 10gm daily. Abrupt discontinuation in such circumstances has led to a withdrawal syndrome similar to alcohol and barbiturate withdrawal. The drug potentiates the activity of inhibitory neurotransmitters glycine and gamma-aminobutyric acid (GABA) and has been shown to act at the GABA-A receptor site.

Characteristics of acute chlormethiazole intoxication

- Sedation leading to coma
- Respiratory depression
- Decreased muscle tone
- Decreased body temperature
- Decreased blood pressure
- Excessive salivation/upper respiratory secretions

- Characteristic (heady 'vegetable' smell) of chlormethiazole on the breath and in gastric lavage fluid
- Poor prognosis in alcoholics/impaired hepatic function.

Treatment of acute intoxication

The following information is for reference only. All cases of substance intoxication should be referred to a National Poisons Information Centre for current treatment advice.

There is no specific antidote to chlormethiazole but early gastric lavage prevents further gastrointestinal absorption. Assisted ventilation is often necessary but the drug is short-acting. Treatment is symptomatic and similar to that for barbiturate intoxication.

Characteristics of chlormethiazole withdrawal syndrome

Excessive prolonged chlormethiazole administration can lead to dependence. Abrupt discontinuation leads to the development of withdrawal symptoms, usually within 24 hours. The syndrome is similar to that associated with barbiturate withdrawal and may vary dramatically in severity from patient to patient and last over a week. It may include the following[101]:

- Uncontrollable tremor
- Excitement/confusion/anxiety/agitation
- Suicidal tendencies
- Hallucinations
- Disorientation of time and place
- Depersonalisation
- Derealisation
- Delusions
- Abdominal pain
- Insomnia
- Seizures
- Sweating

Some individuals may experience residual effects several weeks later including memory impairment, derealisation and depersonalisation.

Flexible chlormethiazole capsule dose — reduction regime[102]

Day	Chlormethiazole capsules/day	Sodium Phenytoin dose
1	30	300mg stat + 100mg tds
2	27	100 mg tds
3	24	100 mg tds
4	21	100 mg tds
5	18	100 mg tds
6	15	50 mg tds
7	12	50 mg tds
8	10	50 mg tds
9	8	50 mg tds
10	6	50 mg bd
11	5	50 mg bd
12	4	50 mg bd
13	3	50 mg od
14	2	50 mg od
15	1	stop
16	0	

Treatment of the withdrawal syndrome

This simply involves reintroduction of chlormethiazole, stabilisation and a gradual discontinuation at a rate tolerated by the client. The Elmdene Alcoholic Treatment and Research Unit, Bexley Hospital, Kent has produced a guide to medical management of chlormethiazole withdrawal in hospitals and copies of this useful document are also available from Astra Pharmaceuticals[102]. It outlines by example a 15 day withdrawal schedule for a client initially taking 30 chlormethiazole capsules daily and advocates antiepileptic cover with phenytoin.

Seizure control may also be achieved using other anticonvulsants and break through seizures controlled by intravenous or rectal diazepam.

Chloral hydrate

Chloral hydrate is a well established hypnotic agent that has been available for clinical use since the 19th century. It was used illicitly for many years and when mixed with alcohol was known as 'knock out drops' or a 'Mickey Finn'. Such mixtures were used to render unsuspecting victims unconscious and some naval recruitment officers of the last century were reputed to have included such mixtures in their armament of 'press gang' techniques. Currently, the drug is licensed for use in both adults and children for short-term treatment of insomnia.

Two chloral derivatives, chloral betaine and triclofos, have been formulated in an attempt to reduce gastric irritancy. Both have similar characteristics to chloral hydrate.

Administration of therapeutic doses quickly produces drowsiness and sedation, followed by sleep within an hour. Blood pressure, respiration and tendon reflexes are all slightly reduced and the hang over effect encountered with many other hypnotics is rare.

Chloral hydrate is a prodrug being quickly metabolised to 2,2,2 trichloroethanol which has a half-life of between 4 and 14 hours. Chronic use of chloral derivatives cause tolerance and physical dependence with an alcohol/barbiturate type withdrawal syndrome. Acute high doses can result in organ damage and potentially fatal intoxication[103].

Characteristics of acute 'chloral' intoxication[103]

Chloral hydrate doses greater than 2gm produce toxicity and fatalities have been reported with doses as low as 1.25 and 3gm. The reported lethal dose is 5 to 10gm but recovery has been reported after ingestion of more than 30gm.

Chloral overdose is manifested in three main ways:

1. CNS depression

2. Skin and mucous membrane corrosion

3. Organ toxicity

Central nervous system depression occurs within 30 minutes of chloral ingestion and is characterised by the following:

- Drowsiness progressing to deep stupor and coma
- Slow/shallow respiration/apnoea
- Lowered body temperature
- Hypotension
- Mottled skin and cyanosis
- Contracted pupils (becoming dilated late)

Death may occur within a few hours or more suddenly due to ventricular arrhythmias and cardiovascular collapse.

The corrosive nature of chloral derivatives causes gastritis, nausea and vomiting. This is particularly marked after ingestion on an empty stomach. However most of the signs and symptoms of this toxic effect are delayed, emerging during the recovery from overdose. They are as follows:

- Haemorrhagic gastritis
- Gastric necrosis
- Enteritis
- Oesophagitis (with strictures)
- Allergic skin reactions (up to 10 days after overdose)

Organ toxicity affects the liver, kidneys and heart. Hepatic cirrhosis with jaundice and nephrotoxicity with albuminurea have been reported. Cardiac toxicity involves the production of abnormal, often pathological heart rhythms. They include ventricular and supraventricular tachyarrhythmias, fibrillations and cardiac arrest. The proposed explanations for the production of such arrhythmias involve the ability of trichloroethanol to release endogenous catecholamines which sensitise the myocardium[103,104].

Treatment of acute intoxication

The following information is for reference only. All cases of acute substance intoxication require referral to a National Poisons Information Centre for current management advice.

Treatment is largely supportive consisting of adequate airways and blood pressure maintenance and assisted respiration where necessary. Other considerations include maintenance of body temperature and prevention of hypoglycaemia secondary to hepatic damage.

Severe intoxication will require active drug removal. Forced diuresis is of limited value. Haemodialysis and haemoperfusion have been used to enhance trichloroethanol clearance in cases of severe intoxication.

Cardiac arrhythmias have been treated with lignocaine,[105,106] but other therapies may be needed if *Torsades de Pointes* occurs.

Multiform ventricular tachycardias resistant to other antiarrhythmics have successfully been treated with beta blockers[107].

Characteristics of chloral hydrate withdrawal syndrome

Chronic use of chloral hydrate may result in tolerance and physical and psychological dependence on the drug. Symptoms of dependence are similar to those of chronic alcoholism and barbiturate dependence and include drowsiness, lethargy, hangover, slurred speech, nystagmus, tremor and incoordination. Gastritis, skin eruptions and renal damage have occurred following prolonged administration.

Abrupt discontinuation of chloral hydrate in a dependent individual can precipitate a withdrawal syndrome similar to that associated with alcohol and barbiturate withdrawal.

It begins with feeling of apprehension and anxiety with muscle weakness, headache, tremors, nausea and vomiting and abdominal cramps. Hypotension and tachycardia are a feature. Convulsions may be delayed but severe, developing into status epilepticus in some cases. Delirium tremens may also be a feature. It is characterised by illusions, hallucinations, further increased confusion and excitement with tremor.

Management of the withdrawal syndrome

Emergence of a withdrawal syndrome can usually be treated by reintroduction of a sedative hypnotic agent followed by a more gradual withdrawal. In the case of chloral hydrate, discontinuation over a 7–10 period would be appropriate. However, as with all cases of successful withdrawal, the rate should be determined by what the client can tolerate.

Chapter 8
VOLATILE ORGANIC
SOLVENTS AND RELATED
SUBSTANCES

Volatile organic solvents generally have few medical uses except for a handful that are used as anaesthetic gases. Those that are misused are found in household items and thus lend themselves to easy acquisition.

Common organic solvents and sources[108,109]	
Butane	Aerosols/lighter fluid
Esters	Marker pens/adhesives
Halons	Fire extinguishers
Ketones	Nail varnish remover
Paraffin	Garages/hardware stores
Petrol	Garages
Tetrachloroethylene	Dry cleaning and stain removing
Trichlorethylene	products. Plaster remover
Toluene	Adhesives/glues
Xylene	

Solvent inhalation is predominantly a pastime of a minority of school children. Since 1985 it has been reported as resulting in over 100 deaths annually which represents about 4% of annual UK adolescent deaths. It is estimated that between 3.5 and 10% of adolescents have experimented with volatile substances and about 1% of adolescents are chronic users.

Methods of administration[108,109]

As the practise suggests, volatile substance inhalation involves the breathing in of vapours/gas from organic solvents and related substances, found in various commercial products. This often involves rebreathing the vapours from a plastic bag, either placed over the mouth or completely over the head. Other methods include inhalation from confined spaces such as under bed covers.

Aerosol propellants can be sprayed directly into the throat. Fumes can be inhaled from solvent soaked clothing e.g. handkerchiefs and scarves.

Effects of acute volatile organic substance inhalation[108]

The first effects of inhalation include euphoria (buzz or rush), excitation (possibly secondary to disinhibition), disinhibition, and heightened emotions and sociability. This is followed by rapidly developing CNS depression, confusion and perceptual disturbances.

Delusions and hallucinations may lead to aggressive or risk-taking behaviour. Further CNS depression leads to ataxia, nystagmus, dysarthria, drowsiness and sedation.

Unconsciousness and coma are accompanied by respiratory depression and occasional seizures. Vomiting, sneezing and coughing are possible as is salivation occurring at any stage of intoxication.

Most importantly, sudden death can occur via various mechanisms and has occurred several hours after the intoxication has apparently subsided.

Deaths related to solvent use[108,109]

Causes of sudden death in cases of solvent use are various and include suffocation, choking, cardiac arrest secondary to vagal stimulation, respiratory depression, trauma and cardiac arrhythmias.

Cardiac arrhythmias account for about half of all volatile substance-related deaths. The heart tissue is sensitised to the effects of noradrenaline and other sympathetic amines. Users who are emotionally or physically stressed are particularly vulnerable and the sensitising effect is still present several hours after using the solvent. If a child is discovered inhaling solvents the situation should be handled calmly and quietly. Once the cardiac arrhythmia has developed, resuscitation attempts are often unsuccessful and each separate episode of solvent use is equally dangerous in this respect.

Anoxia results in nearly a third of deaths. It may be due to the inhalation of vomit whilst unconscious, accidental asphyxiation or respiratory depression. Asphyxiation commonly occurs during the practise of placing a plastic bag over the head and rebreathing solvent fumes. Respiratory depression is a result of progressive central nervous depression. Anoxia also potentiates cardiac arrhythmias.

Cardiac arrest is associated with the administration practise of spraying gas (often butane from pressurised lighter refill cans) directly into the throat. Rapid evaporation of gas from the throat cools the pharynx which in turn stimulates the vagus nerve. This results in slowing the heart beat and can eventually stop the heart altogether.

Trauma results in 2–3% of deaths and includes accidents or suicide. The substance usually associated with trauma is toluene. Why this should be the case is not known.

Treatment of the above potentially fatal complications is standard and may require cardiopulmonary resuscitation or intensive care.

Effects of chronic volatile substance inhalation[110,110,112]

Chronic volatile substance inhalation has been reported to lead to poor concentration, insomnia and nightmares. Other complaints have included perioral eczema, gastrointestinal upset and muscle damage. Organ damage may also be a feature of chronic use.

Damage to organs such as the heart, lungs, liver and kidneys has been associated with toluene, trichloroethane and trichorethylene. Neurological damage has been associated with the inhalation of toluene, N-hexane and methy-n-butyl ketone. Toluene has been reported to cause cerebellar disease and chronic encephalitis whilst the other two are associated with peripheral neuropathy. Chronic petrol inhalation leads to lead and benzene poisoning.

Tolerance and withdrawal

Tolerance develops with regular use and larger amounts of solvent are required to attain the desired effect. Symptoms similar to alcohol withdrawal have been reported following abrupt discontinuation. However, general consensus is that this is very rare and abrupt discontinuation is the best method for stopping solvent use.

Dependence

Solvents have reinforcing properties in animals. However, dependence has not been recognised as a problem. There are no pharmacological measures to deal with chronic solvent use. Abrupt solvent discontinuation is currently acceptable. Abstinence is encouraged by various social and psychological supports in the community.

Chapter 9
ILLICIT DRUG USE IN PREGNANCY

Chronic illicit drug use can reduce female fertility. This is especially true for opioid users who may also experience erratic or absent menstrual periods. However, the belief held by some female users that, while taking drugs they cannot get pregnant, is unfounded. As a result of this and other factors, unplanned pregnancy is not an uncommon event among female illicit drug users. While such a pregnancy may be viewed with ambivalence by the user, it can also present significant difficulties for the attending obstetrician and neonatologist.

The relative risks of illicit drug use in pregnancy are difficult to establish as much information on the subject is anecdotal. Interpretation of pregnancy outcomes are further complicated by the fact that users have erratic life-styles and may expose themselves and the foetus to a variety of different drugs and circumstances during pregnancy. Confounding factors include maternal malnutrition, poor hygiene, fragmented antenatal care and the increased risk of infections associated with intravenous drug administration and promiscuity[113].

The most emotive aspect of illicit drug use in pregnancy is the potential danger to the foetus. While maternal drug use may affect foetal development in several ways, the most feared is probably that of congenital malformations (teratogenesis). Until the publicity surrounding the 'Thalidomide Tragedy' in the late 1950s, the potential for drug-induced malformations was not fully realised. Since that time it has probably been overemphasised. However, first trimester foetal drug exposure can lead directly to congenital malformations. Exposure during the third to eleventh week of pregnancy seems to hold the greatest risk to the foetus in this respect. Despite this fact, the observed incidence of congenital malformations among infants born to illicit drug users is estimated to be about 3% at birth. This compares well with the incidence of major congenital anomalies in the overall neonatal population of between 3–4%[114].

Second and third trimester foetal drug exposure can result in reduced foetal growth and spontaneous abortion. Neonates have been born prematurely, small for gestational age and have demonstrated poor prognostic ratings. Maternal drug use in the third trimester is also associated with neonatal drug intoxication at birth and neonatal withdrawal syndrome. Various medical complications have been reported to be more prevalent in pregnancies associated with concurrent drug use. However, the majority of illicit drug users would appear to give birth to infants that are normal. Indeed a recent report suggested that, in the case of cocaine, its' effects on the foetus have been overemphasised and that this has led to unnecessary terminations[115].

Illicit drug-related complications of pregnancy[116,117,118]

Complications reported in association with concurrent illicit drug use are contained below. Specific drug classes are dealt with separately.

Opioids

Methadone is commonly used in pregnant opioid dependants as a maintenance therapy. It has a very low teratogenic potential. The following has been reported:

- Maternal malnutrition
- Severe sickness
- Hypertensive disease of pregnancy
- Detached placenta
- Spontaneous foetal abortion

- Foetal growth retardation
- Inflamed foetal membranes
- Premature rupture of membranes
- Low birth weights/small heads
- Neonatal meconium staining
- Neonatal hypermagnesaemia
- Neonatal intoxication and withdrawal syndrome

CNS stimulants

These drugs have few medical uses. Appetite suppression is inappropriate in pregnancy as is stimulant maintenance therapy.
Reported problems are as follows:

- Maternal malnutrition
- Hypertensive disease of pregnancy
- Increased maternal mortality
- Detached placenta
- Placental ischaemia
- Spontaneous abortion
- Neonatal cerebral ischaemia
- Congenital malformations
- Low birth weight
- Meconium staining
- Neonatal withdrawal syndrome
- Infant behavioural abnormalities

Barbiturates

Barbiturates have been associated with teratogenesis, post-partum and neonatal haemorrhage. Third trimester exposure may result in neonatal withdrawal syndrome where seizures are a feature. Abrupt maternal barbiturate discontinuation may result in a characteristic withdrawal syndrome.

Volatile organic solvents

Although deliberate exposure during pregnancy is rare, evidence of adverse perinatal outcomes are available.

Petrol inhalation has led to neonatal neurodevelopmental impairment including spastic quadriplegia. Maternal lead poisoning is also a risk.

Toluene has been associated with cerebellar degeneration, cortical atrophy, microcephaly, minor craniofacial and limb defects and growth retardation.

Benzodiazepines

Chronic high doses may lead to intrauterine growth retardation, Floppy Infant Syndrome and neonatal withdrawal syndrome. Congenital malformations have also been reported.

Cannabis

Cannabis has been associated with childhood non-lymphoblastic leukaemia. There have also been conflicting reports concerning gestation length, duration of labour, foetal growth, congenital defects and infant behaviour.

Phencyclidine (PCP)

Most recorded maternal PCP exposures have resulted in few problems for mother or child. Neonatal irritability, jitteriness, hypertoniticity and poor feeding have been reported.

LSD

LSD is usually taken in very small quantities (100–150mcg). Briggs *et al.* conclude that pure LSD is not associated with chromosomal abnormalities, spontaneous abortion or teratogenicity[117]. Early reports of such events involved multi-drug use.

Management of the pregnant illicit drug user

In all cases, it is better to avoid use of medicines in pregnancy unless the benefits of such use outweigh the risks to the foetus and mother. Where illicit drugs are involved, drug discontinuation is advisable especially where there is a higher risk of congenital abnormalities. How the drug is discontinued will depend on the nature of the drug, dependence and withdrawal potential and the risk to the foetus during the discontinuation process.

The department of health has issued brief guidance on the general management of pregnant illicit drug users with particular emphasis on opioid dependence, as this is perceived to be the biggest problem area[116]. However, while antenatal care is available to all pregnant individuals, drug users often make little use of it for various reasons. General attitudes of health care providers can be markedly disapproving of the pregnant user. She is therefore more likely to view antenatal care unfavourably. Shapiro addresses these issues clearly and in some detail, advocating a sensitive antenatal approach[119].

Opioids

Opioid use is associated with nausea and vomiting. Chronic drug use and poor nutrition is often accompanied by cessation of regular menstruation. As a result, pregnant opioid users may not initially be aware of their condition. When they are aware, it is a common response to abruptly discontinue their drug use so as not to harm the baby. Unfortunately, such action can precipitate an acute maternal withdrawal syndrome and is also potentially life-threatening to the foetus.

If the user contacts a medical practitioner it is appropriate to prescribe methadone maintenance therapy, at least temporarily. Liason between the pregnant client's drug workers and the attending clinician is desirable throughout the pregnancy. It is at this time that HIV counselling and subsequent testing if appropriate should take place and decisions made on how to proceed. If the client wishes to continue with the pregnancy early referral to an obstetrician is indicated. Good liaison between obstetric and drug misuser services is desirable. This, coupled with a tolerant, understanding approach will increase the chances of retaining contact with the client and so ensure effective antenatal care.

The obstetrician has several options for managing the client's pregnancy. These include gradual methadone discontinuation conducted either in the community or in hospital, continued methadone maintenance throughout pregnancy, or partial withdrawal followed by low dose methadone maintenance.

Inpatient (hospital)-based methadone discontinuation

Methadone discontinuation is ideally conducted during the second trimester. In this way the risks of premature labour and abortion are minimised. Following the establishment of a stabilising methadone dose, the discontinuation process is more gradual than that undertaken for nonpregnant clients and is anticipated to take about 12 weeks. Dose decrements should be no greater than 5mg per week even at the beginning. Towards the end of the 12 weeks period, dose decrements are likely to be 1 to 2mg, again implemented at approximately weekly intervals. Single or twice daily dose administration is appropriate.

Some workers have implemented methadone discontinuation regimen employing daily dose decrements of 1mg with good success. However this may result in too rapid a withdrawal.

Although the most expensive option, inpatient methadone discontinuation has several advantages over outpatient management. These include the following:

1. Closer foetal and placental monitoring.

2. Closer methadone dose titration against withdrawal symptoms.

3. Higher initial success rate.

4. There is less chance of maternal exposure to illicit opioids and excipients.

5. It provides better care for clients with unstable social

backgrounds.

If complete within 4 to 6 weeks of the birth the effects of neonatal withdrawal syndrome are likely to be minimal.

Outpatient methadone discontinuation

Like impatient discontinuation, the process should take about 12 weeks. Again it is begun ideally in the second trimester. The regimen is similar to that described for the inpatient but obviously there is less flexibility as far as dose titration is concerned.

Outpatient regimen are more suited to those with a stable social background and good support from family and friends.

Partial methadone discontinuation

Another management strategy includes initial methadone stabilisation followed by gradual dose reduction to a new lower dose of 15–20mg per day. This partial discontinuation is performed in a similar manner to full discontinuation until the lower daily dose is achieved.

This approach is more likely to suit clients with a history of high dose chronic opioid use where complete discontinuation may have previously proved unsuccessful. Clients presenting for management beyond the mid-trimester may also be more suitably treated in this fashion. The low methadone dose is less likely to adversely affect the neonate.

Methadone maintenance

Full maintenance is more likely to suit clients who have previously been unsuccessful in methadone or other opioid detoxification. It is more likely to result in acute neonatal intoxication at delivery and a subsequent neonatal withdrawal syndrome.

Other Drugs

Pregnant users of amphetamines, cocaine and other stimulants should be encouraged to stop use abruptly, as should users of psychedelic drugs (LSD, MDMA, MDA), anaesthetic agents and volatile organic substances. All are potentially harmful to the foetus but are not associated with protracted withdrawal syndromes likely to harm the foetus. Maintenance therapy is not appropriate in these circumstances.

Barbiturates, chloral derivatives and chormethiazole should all be withdrawn gradually. This is to avoid the continued potential for harm to the foetus and the barbiturate-alcohol type withdrawal syndrome in both mother and neonate. Too rapid a withdrawal may result in seizures and a withdrawal period of eight to ten days is appropriate. Barbiturate dependent individuals first require conversion of their daily barbiturate intake to a phenobarbitone equivalent (100mg of short-acting barbiturate = 30mg phenobarbitone). The resulting phenobarbitone dose is then reduced on a daily or alternate day basis until complete discontinuation is achieved. This is best illustrated by example[20]:

A drug user taking 900mg of pentobarbitone daily is given 270mg phenobarbitone as the initial daily dose. The proposed reduction regime will then be as follows:

Day	Daily Phenobarbitone dosing schedule
1	90mg tds
2	90mg tds
3	60mg tds
4	60mg tds
5	60mg bd
6	60mg bd
7	30mg bd
8	30mg bd
9	stop

This is a similar approach to that outlined in the 'barbiturates section' and is to be considered a guide.

Benzodiazepines also need to be withdrawn gradually. Therapeutic doses can usually be discontinued on an outpatient basis over a four week period[20]. Some clients require longer, and others may not achieve abstinence. Benzodiazepines taken in doses equivalent to 60mg diazepam or more per day require impatient management to avoid the increased risk of fitting.

Banks and Waller advocate a detoxification time scale of one to two weeks[120]. However this is a very short time period and effective benzodiazepine withdrawal may require twelve weeks or more[73,74,80,81].

Chapter 10
NEWBORN INFANTS OF DRUG-DEPENDENT MOTHERS

Maternal drug use in the third trimester of pregnancy is likely to result in neonatal intoxication and in the case of narcotic agents (eg. opioids, benzodiazepines, barbiturates, CNS stimulants) a neonatal withdrawal syndrome may occur.

As methadone maintenance is a common management strategy for pregnant opioid dependants, neonatal methadone intoxication and neonatal opioid withdrawal syndrome are most commonly encountered.

Newborn infants of mothers dependent on opioids[113,121,122,123]

Newborn infants of opioid-dependent women may initially demonstrate opioid intoxication resulting in respiratory depression. Some time later, they may present with a withdrawal syndrome. Its severity may not correlate well with the extent of maternal opioid usage or duration of exposure, and withdrawal onset will depend in part on the substance used.

Subacute methadone withdrawal has been reported three to six **months** after birth in some infants[113], but other experts question the validity of these claims.

Neonatal opioid intoxication

Ideally, this is managed in the hospital setting. Intoxication is characterised by depressed respiration and sedation despite adequate cardiac output and the initial establishment of breathing.

Treatment with naloxone

The following is for reference only as practices vary between neonatal units. It is usual to establish an adequate airway in the apnoeic infant and then to use naloxone. The data sheet recommends a dose of 0.01 mg/kg administered intravenously for opioid-induced respiratory depression. Such doses are repeated at 2 to 3 minute intervals if necessary[3]. The effect is immediate but is only sustained for about 30 minutes. Administration via this route is useful diagnostically but repeated IV injections are inconvenient. A single 200mcg intramuscular dose can be used. It has a slower onset of action but can last up to 18 to 24 hours. This is probably due to a depot effect created at the site of injection. Intramuscular doses of 100mcg are used for babies less than 2kg in weight.

Characteristics of the neonatal (opioid) withdrawal syndrome

The signs and symptoms of neonatal opioid withdrawal syndrome are usually non-specific and can apply to the infants of mothers who have regularly taken CNS stimulants, opioids and other sedative/hypnotic drugs. The condition is also known as neonatal narcotic syndrome and neonatal withdrawal syndrome. Onset of withdrawal symptoms will be delayed with long-acting opioids, and the duration of the syndrome will be prolonged.

| Heroin (diamorphine) | Onset within 72 hours. Duration approximately 7 days. |
| Methadone | Onset between 4 and 12 days. Duration — 2 to 4 weeks. |

Neonates may demonstrate the following[113,121,122,123,124,125,126]

- Irritability
- Sleeplessness
- Shrill crying
- Hypertonia with intermittent hypotonia
- Tremor and shaking
- Sweating/yawning
- Nasal stuffiness
- Sneezing
- Spitting
- Continuous purposeless sucking
- Vomiting
- Frequent loose stools
- Raised magnesium levels
- Convulsion (more frequent with methadone withdrawal)
- Low size and birth weight

Treatment of neonatal withdrawal syndrome

The withdrawal syndrome of neonates born to opioid-dependent mothers (and those dependent on CNS stimulant and narcotic agents) can be a self-limiting condition which subsides uneventfully after several days without a need for definitive therapy. Although the narcotic withdrawal syndrome is not associated with significantly increased mortality, it has been suggested that infants with progressive irritability, feeding difficulties and weight loss exceeding 10% of birth weight will benefit from drug therapy[123]. It is most likely that such neonates will be treated in a hospital environment. Measures such as tight swaddling, frequent feeding and minimal photic stimulation have met with mixed success.

General management includes regular and frequent feeds to ensure adequate hydration in the face of diarrhoea and vomiting.

The attending clinician may use one of a variety of possible drug treatments to alleviate the infant's discomfort depending upon the current unit practices.

Regimens that have been used to treat neonatal withdrawal syndrome[126]

Drug	Regimen	Notes
Camphorated Opium tincture	0.2–0.7ml 3 hourly for 1 week. Then gradually withdraw	Camphor stimulates CNS. Benzoic acid displaces bilirubin. Contains noscapine. Not recommended
Diluted tincture of opium	0.4mg morphine 4 hourly for 1–2 weeks, then gradually withdraw	Contains noscapine. Not recommended
Methadone	0.25–0.5mg 4–12 hourly gradually reducing over several weeks	
Diazepam*	1–2mg IM 8 hourly until symptoms are controlled then reduce. Treat for 1 week or 3.6mg/kg/day orally in 3 divided doses	May cause respiratory depression if given with barbiturates. Does not modify diarrhoea
Chlorpromazine	2–3mg/kg/day in 4 divided doses for 5–10 days then gradually withdraw after 2–3 weeks	

Drug	Regimen	Notes
Phenobarbitone	5–10mg/kg/day in 3–4 divided doses for 10 days then gradually withdraw	Controls seizures and improves irritability and insomnia. Does not control diarrhoea
Clonidine	Challenge dose 0.5–1mcg/kg then 3–4mcg/kg/day in 4 divided doses	For opioid withdrawal. (Two infant study). Treatment given for 10 and 16 days. Not routinely recommended
* The BNF advises that intramuscular diazepam should only be administered where oral or IV routes are unavailable. Others recommend diazepam is administered only by oral or slow IV routes[124].		

Some practitioners consider that it is necessary and desirable to fully involve the mother in the withdrawal process. Full explanation is required to avoid undue distress to the family during the withdrawal period

REFERENCES

1. McEvoy GK ed (1991) Opiate agonists general statement. In: *American Hospital Formulary Service 91*. American Society of Hospital Pharmacists. 1145–9

2. Reynolds JEF ed (1989) Opiate analgesics. In: Martindale. *The Extra Pharmacopoeia 29th edn*. The Pharmaceutical Press: 1294–1321

3. Narcan and Narcan (1991) Neonatal (1991). In: *ABPI Data Sheet Compendium*. Datapharm Publications, London: 433–44.

4. McKinney *et al* (1988) Drug abuse. In: Young LY, Koda-Kimble MA eds. *Applied Therapeutics, 4th edn*. Applied Therapeutics, Washington: 1277–312

5. Greighton FJ, Ghodse AH (1989) Naloxone applied to the conjunctiva as a test for physical opiate dependence. *Lancet* i: 748

6. Goulding JA *et al* (1987) Poisoning with drugs and chemical substances. In: Weatherall DJ, Ledingham JGG, Warrell DA eds. *Oxford Textbook of Medicine, 2nd edn*. Oxford Medical Publishers: 6.23–6.24

7. Mitcheson M (1987) Drug addiction. In: Weatherall DJ, Ledingham JGG, Warrell DA eds. *Oxford Textbook of Medicine 2nd edn*. Oxford Medical Publishers: 25.25–25.30

8. Charney DS *et al* (1986) The combined use of clonidine and naltrexone as a rapid, safe and effective treatment of abrupt withdrawal from methadone. *Am J Psychiatry* **143**: 831–7

9. Gossop M (1987) What is the most effective way to treat opiate addiction? *Br J Hosp Med* **38**: 161

10. Brewer C (1988) Methadone maintenance: Theory and Practice. *Pharm J* **241**: 322–4

11.   Gossop M (1988) Clonidine and the treatment of opiate withdrawal syndrome. *Drug Alcohol Depend* 21: 253–9

12.   Gossop M (1978) A review of the evidence for methadone maintenance as a treatment for narcotic addiction. *Lancet* ii: 812–6

13.   Prasad AB ed (1992) Antihypertensive therapy. In: *The British National Formulary No 24*. BMA and RPSGB: 84

14.   Washton AM, Resruck RB, Gretchen G (1983) Opiate withdrawal using lofexidine. A clonidine analogue with fewer side-effects. *J Clin Psychiatry* 44: 335–7

15.   ABPI (1994) Britlofex tablets, 0.2mg. In: *ABPI Data Compendium 1994–95*. Datapharm Publications, Ltd. London: 319

16.   Gold MS, Pottash AC, Sweeney DR, Extein I, Annitto WJ (1981) Opiate detoxification with lofexidine. *Drug Alcohol Depend* 8: 307–15

17.   Pharmaceutical Journal (1991) Clonidine in drug withdrawal. *Pharm J* 247: 536

18.   Ternes JW, O'Brian CP (1990) The opioids: Abuse liability and treatments for dependence. *Adv Alcohol Drug Substance Abuse* 9: 27–47

19.   Weber R *et al* (1990) Progression of HIV infection in misusers of injected drugs who stop injecting or follow a programme of maintenance treatment with methadone. *Br Med J* 301: 1362–5

20.   Marks JA, Palombella A (1990) Prescribing smokable drugs. *Lancet* 335: 864

21.   Skidmore CA *et al* (1990) After the epidemic: follow up study of HIV seroprevalence and changing patterns of drug use. *Br Med J* 300: 219–23

22.   Bloor RN, Smalldridge NJF (1990) Intravenous use of slow release morphine sulphate tablets. *Br Med J* 300: 640–1

23.   Ohaf H *et al* (1990) Deaths of heroin addicts starting on a methadone maintenance programme. *Lancet* 335: 108

24.   Dole VP (1989) Methadone treatment and the Aquired Immunodeficiency Syndrome Epidemic. *J Am Med Assoc* 262: 1681–2

25.   Johnson RE *et al* (1989) Use of buprenorphine in the treatment of opiate addiction, I. Physiological and behavioural effects during a rapid dose introduction. *Clin Pharmacol Therap* **46**: 335–43

26.   Fundala PJ *et al* (1990) Use of buprenorphine in the treatment of opiate addiction, II. Physiological and behavioural effects of daily and alternate day administration and abrupt withdrawal. *Clin Pharmacol Therap* **47**: 525–34

27.   Gawin FH, Ellinwood EH (1988) Cocaine and other stimulants. *N Engl J Med* **318**: 1173–82

28.   Miller NS, Gold MS, Millman RB (1989) Cocaine: General characteristics, abuse and addiction. *N Y State J Med* **89**: 390–4

29.   Council on Scientific Affairs (1978) Council Report. Clinical Aspects of Amphetamine Abuse. *J Am Med Assoc* **240**: 2317–22

30.   *Cocaine/Amphetamine. Toxbase* (1992). Primary data base of the UK National Poisons Information Service, Edinburgh Royal Infirmary

31.   Strang J, Edwards Griffith (1989) Cocaine and crack. *Br Med J* **299**: 337–8

32.   Taylor WA, Gold MS (1990) Pharmacological approaches to the treatment of cocaine dependence. Addiction Medicine (special issue) *West J Med* **152**: 573–7

33.   Lacombe S *et al* (1991) Pharmacological treatment of cocaine abuse. *DICP Ann Pharmacother* **25**: 818–23

34.   Opie LH, Singh BN (1987) Calcium channel antagonists. In: Opie LH ed. *Drugs for the Heart 2nd edn*. Grune and Statton: 34–53

35.   Regnolds JEF ed. (1989) Index to clinical uses. In: Martindale, *The Extra Pharmacopoeia 29th edn*. The Pharmaceutical Press: 1681–99

36.   Halikas J *et al* (1989) Carbamazepine for cocaine addiction. *Lancet* **ii**: 623

37.   Brewer C (1989) Cocaine and crack (communications). *Br Med J* **229**: 792

38.   Stockley IH ed (1991) *Drug Interactions 2nd edn*. Blackwell Scientific: 549–50

39. Berger P, Gawin F, Kosten TR (1989) Treatment of cocaine abuse with mazindol. *Lancet* **i:** 283

40. Institute for the Study of Drug Dependence (1992) *Isdd Drug notes 8. Ecstasy*. Institute for the Study of Drug Dependence, London

41. Shulgin AT (1986) The background and chemistry of MDMA. *J Psychoactive Drugs* **18:** 291–304

42. Hayner GN, McKinney H (1986) MDMA. The dark side of ecstasy. *J Psychoactive Drugs* **18:** 341

43. Beck J, Morgan PA (1986) Designer Drug Confusion : A focus on MDMA. *J Death Dying* **16:** 287–302

44. Climco RP, Rohrick H, Sweeny DR, Al-Razi J (1987) Ecstasy — a review of MDMA and MDA. *Int J Psychiatry Med* **16:** 359–71

45. McGuire P, Fahy T (1991) Chronic paranoid psychosis after misuse of MDMA. *Br Med J* **302:** 697

46. Dowling GP, McDonough ET, Rost RO (1987) Eve and Ecstasy : a report of five deaths associated with use of MDEA and MDMA. *J Am Med Assoc* **257:** 1615–17

47. Suarez RV, Riemersma R (1988) 'Ecstasy' and sudden cardiac death. *Am J Forensic Med Pathol* **9:** 339–41

48. Fahal IH, Sallomi DF, Vaqoob M, Bell GM (1992) Acute renal failure after ecstasy. *Br Med J* **305:** 29

49. Foley RJ, Kapatkin K, Verani R, Weinman EJ (1984) Amphetamine — induced acute renal failure. *South Med J* **77:** 258–9

50. Henry JA (1992) Ecstasy and the dance of death. *Br Med J* **305:** 5–6

51. Weil AT (1976) 'The love drug'. *J Psychedelic Drugs* **8:** 336

52. Dukes MNG (1988) Drugs of abuse. In: Dukes MNG ed. *Meyler's side-effects of Drugs. 11th edn*. Elsevier: 77-89

53. Kulig K (1990) LSD. *Emerg Med Clin North Am* **8:** 551–8

54. Jaffe JH (1985) Drug addiction and drug abuse. In: Goodman LS, Gilman AG eds. *The Pharmacological Basis of Therapeutics. 7th edn*. Macmillian: 561–5

55. Miller PL, Gay GR, Ferris KC, Anderson S (1992) Treatment of acute, adverse psychedelic reactions: 'I've tripped and can't get down'. *J Psychoactive Drugs* **24**(3): 277–9

56. Jacobs MR, Fehr KO'B eds. (1987) Phencyclidine. In: *Drugs and Drugs of Abuse 2nd edn*. Addiction Research Foundation: 433–41

57. Shapiro H (1992) *Ketamine*. Fact sheet. Institute for the Study of Drug Dependence

58. Ellenhorn MJ, Barceloux DG eds. (1987) Phencyclidine. In: *Medical Toxicology, Diagnosis and Treatment of Human Poisoning*. Elsevier Publisher: 764–77

59. Shaffer LL (1974) Ketamine. *J Am Med Assoc* **229**: 763

60. Rainey JM, Crowder MK (1974) Ketamine or Phencyclidine. *J Am Med Assoc* **230**: 824

61. Bazire S (1991) Psychotropics in problem areas. In: *Psychotropic Aide Memoire. 10th edn*. Hellesdon Hospital, Norwich: 6–7

62. Dale JR, Appelbe GE eds (1989) Misuse of Drugs Act 1971. In: *Pharmacy Law and Ethics, 4th edn*. The Pharmaceutical Press: 151–78

63. Institute for the Study of Drug Dependence (1992) I*sdd Drug notes 3. Cannabis*. Institute for the Study of Drug Dependence

64. The Advisory Council on the Misuse of Drugs. *Report of the Expert Council on the Effects of Cannabis Use*. Home Office, London

65. Ashton CH (1987) Cannabis: Dangers and possible uses. *Br Med J* **294**: 141–2

66. Teggin AF, Bewley TH (1979) Withdrawal treatment for barbiturate dependence. *Practice of Medicine* **223**: 106–7

67. McEvoy GK ed (1992) Barbiturates. In: *AHFS Drug Information 92*. American Hospital Formulary Service. American Society of Hospital Pharmacists: 1317–30

68. Meredith TJ, Vale JA eds (1981) Poisoning due to hypnotics, sedatives, tranquillizers and anticonvulsants. In: *Poisoning Diagnosis and Treatment 1st edn*. Update Books: 84,85

69. Reynolds EF ed (1989) Anxiolytics, sedatives hypnotics and

neuroleptics. In: Martindale. *The Extra Pharmacopoeia 29th edn.* The Pharmaceutical Press: 706–76

70.   Buchanan JF *et al* (1992) Drug abuse. In: Koda-Kimble MA, Young LY eds. *Applied Therapeutics. The clinical use of drugs. 5th edn.* Applied Therapeutics: 59–10,11

71.   Lader M (1989) Benzodiazepines in profile. *Prescriber's J* 29: 12–17

72.   Crismon ML, Jann MW (1988) Anxiety and Insomnia. In: Koda-Kimble MA, Young LY eds. *The clinical use of drugs 4th edn.* Applied Therapeutics: 1155–9

73.   Lader N, Morton S (1991) Benzodiazepine problems. *Br J Addict* 86: 823–8

74.   Ashton H (1989) Risks of dependence on benzodiazepine drugs: A major problem of long-term treatment. *Br Med J* 298: 103–4

75.   Prasad AB ed. (1992) Emergency treatment of poisoning. In: *British National Formulary 24th edn.* BMA and RPSGB: 15–22

76.   McEvoy GK ed (1992) Benzodiazepines. In: *AHFS Drug Information 92.* American Hospital Formulary Service. American Society of Hospital Pharmacists: 1330–54

77.   Brogden RN, Goa LK (1991) Flumazenil. A reappraisal of its pharmacological properties and therapeutic efficacy as a benzodiazepine antagonist. *Drugs* 42: 1061–89

78.   Burr W, Sandham P, Judd A (1989) Death after flumazenil. *Br Med J* 298: 1713

79.   Lim AG (1989) Death after flumazenil. *Br Med J* 299: 858–9

80.   Higgitt AC, Lader MH, Fonagy P (1985) Clinical management of benzodiazepine dependence. *Br Med J* 291: 688–90

81.   Tyrer P (1989) Risks of dependence on benzodiazepine drugs: the importance of patient selection. *Br Med J* 298: 102–5

82.   Lader MH, Olande DA (1987) A comparison of buspirone and placebo in relieving benzodiazepine withdrawal symptoms. *J Clin Psychopharmacol* 7: 11–5

83.   Lader MH, Petursson H (1981) Withdrawal from long-term benzodiazepine treatment. *Br Med J* 283: 643–5

84. Joughin N, Tata P, Collins M, Hooper C, Falkowski J (1991) Inpatient withdrawal from long-term benzodiazepine use. *Br J Addict* **86**: 449–55

85. Finley PR, Nolan PE (1989) Precipitation of benzodiazepine withdrawal following sudden discontinuation of midazolam. *DICP Ann Pharmacother* **23**: 151–2

86. Northern Regional Health Authority (1985) *Benzodiazepine dependence and withdrawal — an update.* Drug Newsletter No 31

87. Bazire S (1991) Further information on some psychiatric illnesses and conditions. In: *Psychotropic Aide Memoire, 10th edn*. Hellesdon Hospital, Norwich. 64–9

88. Bazire S (1991) Dosage Equivalents. In: *Psychotropic Aide Memoire, 10th edn*. Hellesdon Hospital, Norwich: 25

89. Taylor D (1989) Guidelines for withdrawing benzodiazepines. *Br J Pharmaceut Pract* **11**: 106–10

90. Prasad AB ed (1992) Drugs acting on the central nervous system. In: *British National Formulary, 24th edn*. BMA and RPSGB: 138–98

91. Klein E, Uhde TW (1986) Preliminary evidence for the utility of carbamazepine in alprazolam withdrawal. *Am J Psychiatry* **143**: 235–8

92. Ashton H (1984) Benzodiazepine withdrawal : An unfinished story. *Br Med J* **288**: 1135–40

93. Bazire S (1991) Benzodiazepine dependence and withdrawal. In: *Psychotropic Aide Memoire, 10th edn*. Hellesdon Hospital, Norwich: 6–7.

94. Savic I, Wilden L, Stone-Elander S (1991) Feasibility of reversing benzodiazepine tolerance with flumazenil. *Lancet* **337**: 133–7

95. Stark C, Sykes R, Mullin P (1987) Temazepam abuse. *Lancet* **ii**: 802–3

96. Blair SD, Holcumbe C, Coombes EN, O'Malley MK (1991) Leg Ischaemia secondary to non-medical injection of temazepam. *Lancet* **338**: 1393

97. Scott N *et al* (1992) Intra-arterial temazepam. *Br Med J* **304**: 1630

98.   Inness CF, Cotter JC, Davies P, Wood N (1992) Misuse of temazepam. *Br Med J* **305**: 823

99.   Fox R, Beeching NJ, Morrison C, Ruben S, Garvey T (1992) Misuse of temazepam. *Br Med J* **305**: 252

100.   Ruben S, Morrison CL (1992) Temazepam misuse in a group of injecting drug users. *Br J Addict* **87**: 1392

101.   Hession MA, Verma S, Bhakta KGM (1979) Dependence on chlormethiazole and effects of its withdrawal. *Lancet* **i**: 953–4

102.   Majumdar SK (1989) *Medical Management of Chlormethiazole (Heminevrin) Withdrawal in Hospital*. Bexley Health Authority, Bexley Hospital, Old Bexley Lane, Bexley, Kent

103.   Seyffart G (1983) Chloral hydrate and related drugs. In: Haddad LM, Winchester JF eds. *Clinical Management of Poisoning and Drug Overdose*. W B Saunders, Philadephia, London: 80–1, 96–9

104.   Gerretsen M, de Groot G, Van Heijst ANP, Maes RAA (1979) Chloral hydrate poisoning : its mechanism and therapy. *Vet Hum Toxicol* **21**(suppl): 53–6

105.   Marshall AJ (1977) Cardiac arrhythmias caused by chloral hydrate. *Br Med J* **2**: 994

106.   Wiseman HM, Hampel G (1978) Cardiac arrhythmias due to chloral hydrate poisoning. *Br Med J* **2**: 960

107.   Bowyer K, Glasser SP (1980) Chloral hydrate overdose and cardiac arrhythmias. *Chest* **77**: 232

108.   Wills S (1993) Volatile substance abuse. *Pharm J* **250**: 381–3

109.   Ashton CH (1990) Solvent abuse. *Br Med J* **300**: 135–6

110.   McLeod AA, Marjot R, Monaghan MJ, Hugh-Jones P, Jackson G (1987) Chronic cardiac toxicity after inhalation of 1,1,1-trichloroethane. *Br Med J* **294**: 727–9

111.   Wiseman MN, Banim S (1987) Glue sniffers heart? *Br Med J* **294**: 739

112.   Day RE, Oliver JS, Lush M, Watson JM (1981) Solvent encephalopathy. *Br Med J* **283**: 663–5

113.   O'Connor MC (1987) Drugs of abuse in pregnancy — An overview. *Med J Aust* **147**: 180–3

114. Merck, Sharp and Dohme (1987) Congenital abnormalities. In: Berkow R ed. The *Merck Manual of Diagnosis and Therapy, 15th edn*. Merck, Sharp and Dohme: 1923–63.

115. Koren G *et al* (1989) Bias against the null hypothesis: The reproductive hazards of cocaine. *Lancet* **ii**: 1440–2

116. Department of Health (1991) *Drug Misuse and Dependence. Guidelines on Clinical Manangement*. Department of Health, Scottish Office, Home and Health Department, Welsh Office. HMSO, London

117. Oppenheimer E (1991) Alcohol and drug misuse among women — an overview. *Br J Psychiatry* **(suppl 10)**: 36–44

118. Briggs GG, Freeman RK, Yaffe SJ eds. (1990) *Drugs in Pregnancy and Lactation. 3rd edn*. Williams and Wilkins. London

119. Shapiro H (1992) Drugs, pregnancy and childcare. A guide for professional, 2nd edn. Institute for the study of drug dependence

120. Banks A, Waller T (1988) *Drug Misuse: A Practical Handbook for GPs*. Blackwell Scientific/Institute for the Study of Drug Dependence

121. Caviston P *et al* (1987) Pregnancy and Opiate Addiction. *Br Med J* **295**: 285–6

122. Klenka HM (1986) Babies born in a district general hospital to mothers taking heroin. *Br Med J* **293**: 745–6

123. Blinick G *et al* (1976) Drug addiction in pregnancy and the neonate. *Am J Obs/Gynae* **125**: 135–42

124. Roberts RJ ed (1984) Fetal and Infant Intoxication. In: *Drug Therapy in Infants*. W B Saunders: 340–1

125. North Western Regional Drug Information Service (1986) *Managing the Pregnant Drug Addict*. Current Topics No. 85: 1–2

126. West Midlands Drug Information Serivce (1983) Drug dependence in pregnancy. *Drug Inform Bull*: 13–7

Index

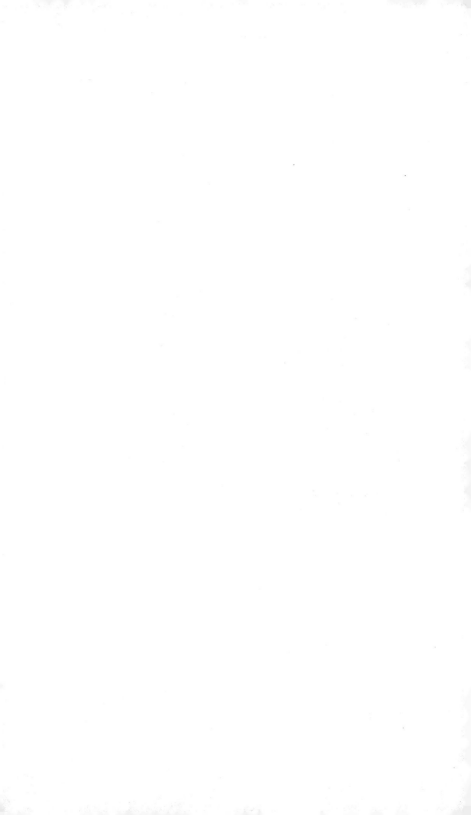

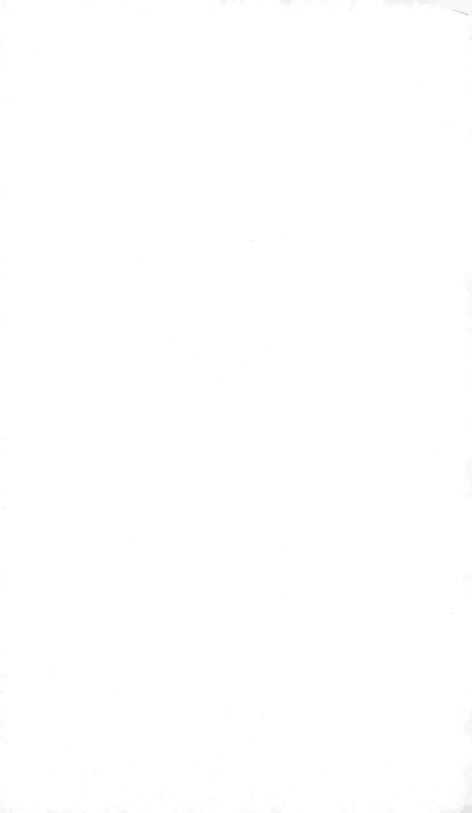

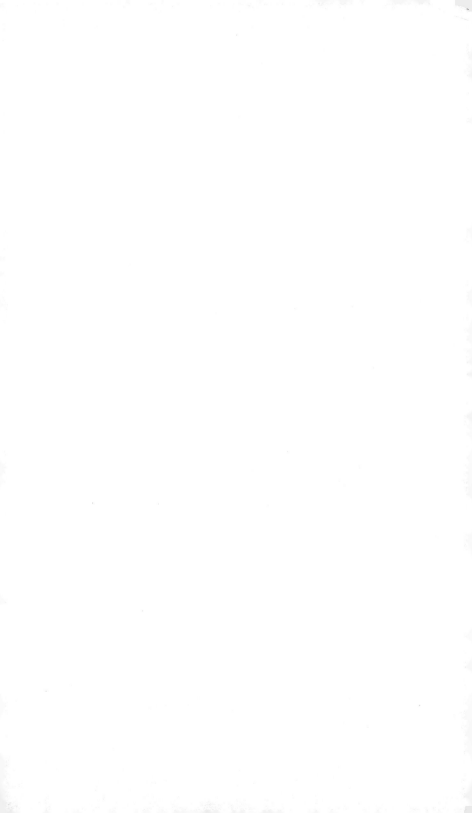